KV-193-090

Lynn Richa...

FIRST LOVE FIRST SEX

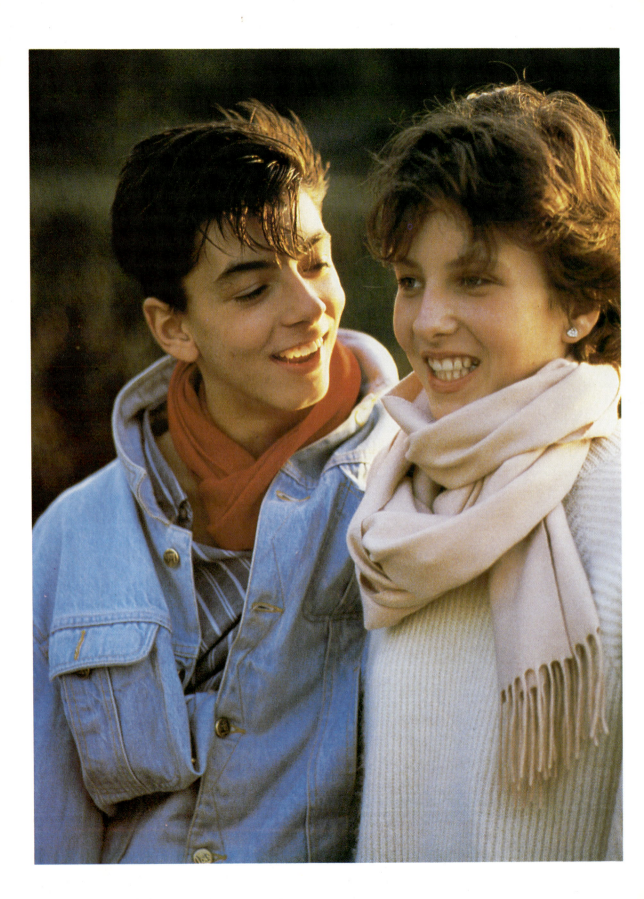

FIRST LOVE FIRST SEX

A practical guide to relationships

by

Kaye Wellings

Recommended
by the
Family Planning
Association

Introduction by
Dr Michael V. Smith

THORSONS PUBLISHING GROUP
Wellingborough · New York

This book was devised and produced by Multimedia Publications (UK) Ltd.

First published in Great Britain in 1986 by Thorsons Publishing Group Ltd, Denington Estate, Wellingborough, Northants NN8 2RQ.

Text © The Family Planning Association 1986
Compilation © Multimedia Publications (UK) Ltd
Photographs and illustrations © Multimedia Publications (UK) Ltd 1986

Editors **Jeff Groman, Anne Cope, Caroline Morrow Brown**
Assistant editor **Andie Oppenheimer**
Production **Karen Bromley**
Design and Art Direction **Terry Allen**
Illustrations **Shari Peacock, Erroll Watson**

British Library Cataloguing in Publication Data

Wellings, Kaye and The Family Planning Association

First Love, First Sex
1. Sex instruction for youth.
I. Title   II. Family Planning Association.
306.7'024055   HQ35

ISBN 0-7225-1233-3

All rights reserved. No part of this publication may be reproduced, stored in a retrieval system, or transmitted in any form or by any means without the prior permission in writing of the publisher and copyright holders, nor be otherwise circulated in any form of binding or cover other than that in which it is published and without a similar condition including this condition being imposed on the subsequent purchaser.

Origination by The Clifton Studio Ltd, London
Typesetting by Keene Graphics Ltd, London
Printed and bound in Spain by Cayfosa. Barcelona. Dep. Leg. B-3801-1986

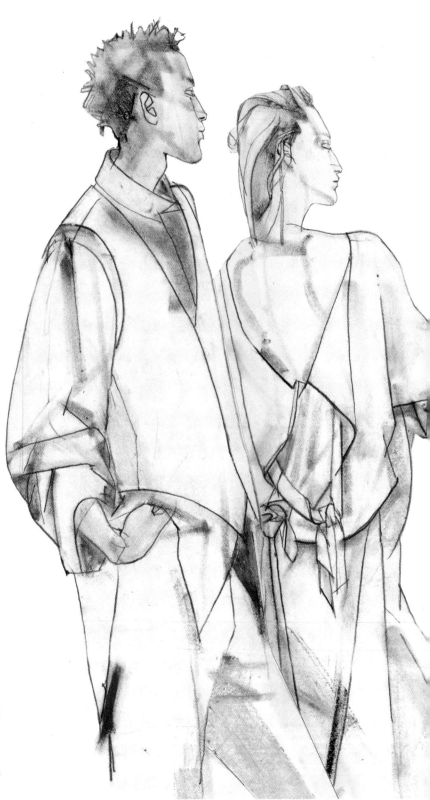

Contents

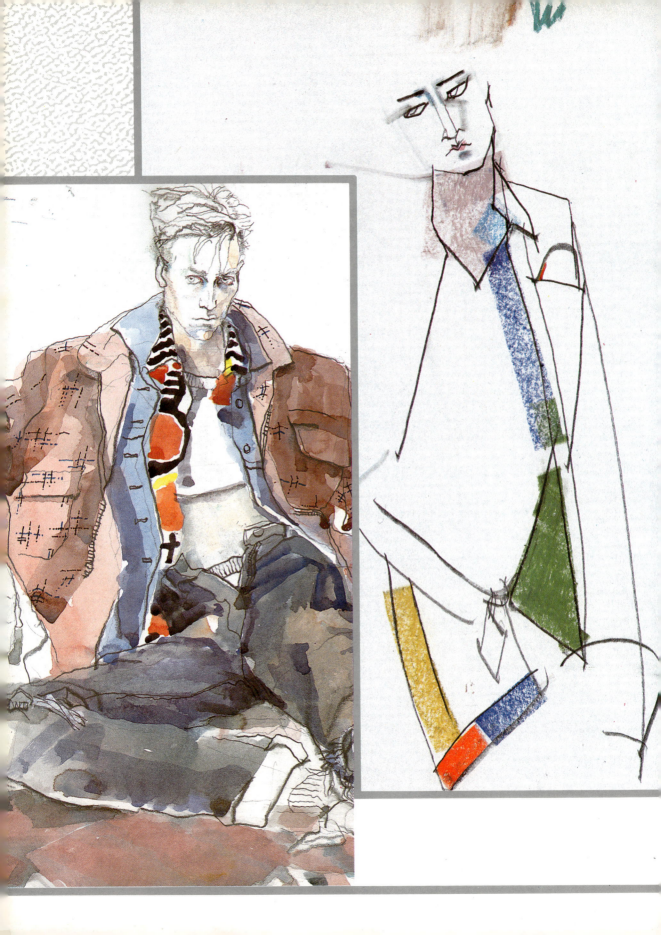

Introduction

by Dr Michael V. Smith
Honorary Chief Medical Officer, Family Planning Association

First love and first sex matter immensely. Our first experiences of both can colour our attitudes and frame our feelings for the rest of our lives. But how well are we prepared for these events?

If our earliest emotional and sexual encounters are enjoyable and rewarding, we feel confident and positive about the future. We are better able to give and to share, to weather the bad times as well as the fun times, and to grow as people.

But a disastrous first love affair or an acutely embarrassing incident at the start of our sexual lives can smoulder and go on hurting for years. It can muddy our expectations and our behaviour, and actually damage our ability to form happy relationships.

What is it about love and sex — two very normal and necessary pursuits — that puts them in the 'handle with care' category? Mainly the fact that we give them such a large space in our lives. They're two of the most potent words in the human language, and bring out our most intense feelings. Without them the world would be a very cold and empty place.

Since the beginning of recorded time, love and sex have been centre stage; wars have raged, kingdoms collapsed, dynasties fallen . . . all for love and the act of sex. Throughout the ages, art, sculpture, music and literature have paid homage to the surging emotions aroused by love and sex. Our pop songs, films, plays, advertisements, books and magazines — and the multinational industries that thrive because of them — circle around the subject of sex like moths around a bright flame.

But when it comes to talking honestly about our feelings and our physical urges, many of us are bashful. So, how are we supposed to find out about the essential facts? How are we supposed to navigate without a map?

If it were easy to talk frankly and openly about love and sex, most of my work as a radio doctor and magazine 'agony uncle' would be unnecessary. As it is, the airwaves tingle and the mailbag bulges with people's sexual and emotional problems — people of all ages and backgrounds, problems of every possible shape, size and variety.

Most of us grow up expecting love, romance and rewarding personal relationships. Nothing wrong in that. These are natural desires, and we feel them most keenly when we are young. We're eager to drink in all that life and love can offer! But being eager for experience isn't the same as being prepared for it.

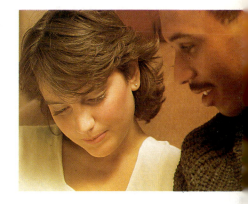

Personally I don't believe that young people today have 'never had it so good'. Certainly there are more options available, but in general anyone growing up today has more pressures to contend with than previous generations ever had. The world is moving very fast, perhaps too fast. There is not much time to stop and consider the real needs of young people. Result: you can find yourself facing life without understanding the facts, let alone the feelings; trying to reach emotional and sexual maturity against a background of too little information and too much disapproval.

The majority of young people in Western societies are becoming sexually active earlier and marrying later. This often means that they have a series of fairly stable but non-permanent relationships before they marry and settle down. How can these relationships be made mutually rewarding? How do you strike a balance between having sexual freedom and being a caring and responsible human being? How do you cope with the difficult issues — embarrassment, shaky self-image, infatuation, jealousy, contraception, sexual health, saying 'no', saying 'yes', saying 'goodbye' — in an appropriate and sensitive way?

This is a book that aims to help young people answer some of these questions for themselves. In order to make sure that the right questions were asked, Kaye Wellings talked to lots of people in their teens and early twenties about what they wanted to know and what they felt. Theirs are the voices that feature throughout this book, and they reflect all kinds of experience — being in love and out of love, being at the beginning and at the end of a sexual relationship, being sexually turned on and turned off, being compatible and incompatible, being happy and being miserable.

First Love, First Sex deals honestly with facts *and* feelings, because both are important. It doesn't hand out rules engraved on tablets of stone, and it doesn't give guarantees — emotional maturity is understanding that life does not come with guarantees. But it is a survival guide. It points out many of the pitfalls and many of the pleasures. It's a book I thoroughly recommend to all young people, and indeed to all those who believe, as I do, that when it comes to love and sex we all have more to learn.

HOW CAN YOUNG PEOPLE TODAY COPE WITH THE DIFFICULT ISSUES OF EMBARRASSMENT, SHAKY SELF-IMAGE, INFATUATION, JEALOUSY, CONTRACEPTION, SAYING 'YES', SAYING 'NO', SAYING 'GOODBYE', IN AN APPROPRIATE AND SENSITIVE WAY?

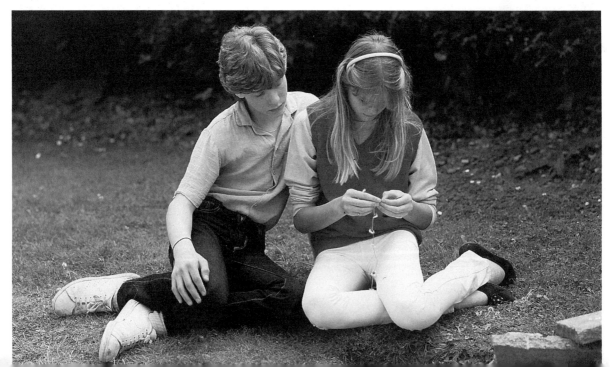

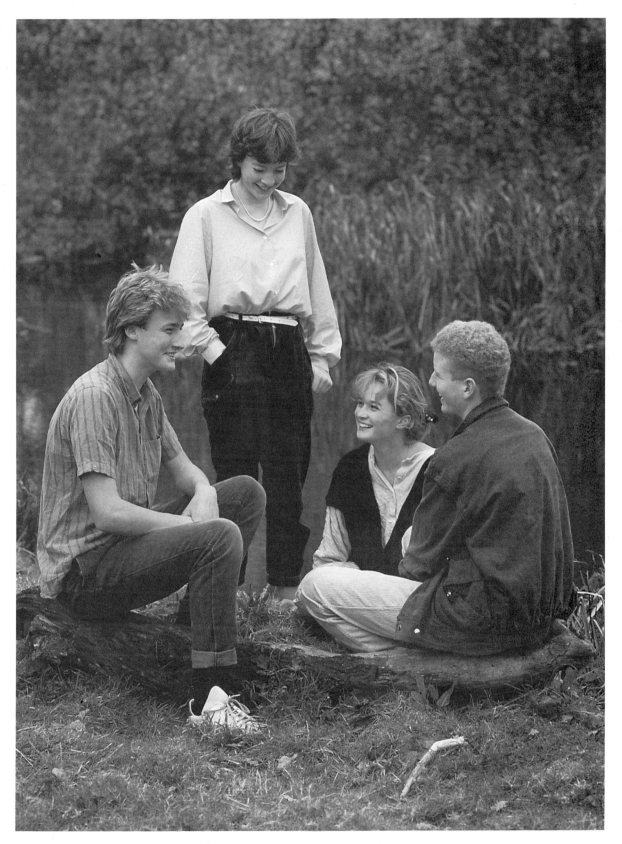

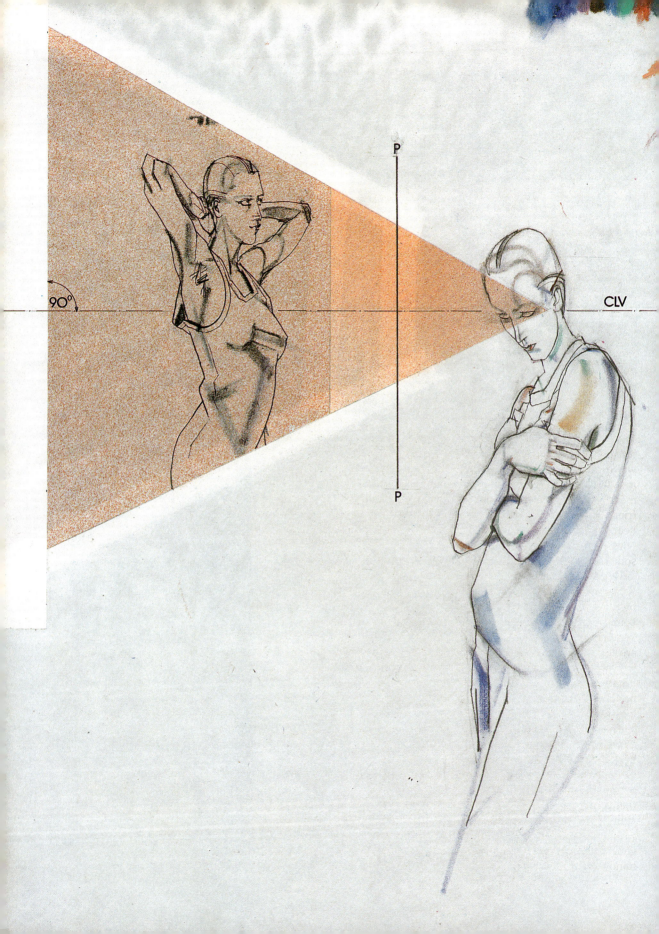

90°

P

P

CLV

1 Presenting yourself

In our society we are quite literally bombarded with images of beautiful men and women every day of our lives — in TV series and commercials, in newspaper and magazine advertisements. An ordinary mortal, it seems, can't sell *anything!* And magazine articles constantly drive home how important it is to look good —'How to have a better body/more sex appeal/ clearer skin/shinier hair'.

First impressions

The plain truth is, of course, that it *does* help to be attractive. Initially we *do* judge people on what they look like. It may seem unfair, but looks are all we've got to go on to begin with. It is said that the most crucial period in a meeting between two people is the first five minutes. During that time we make snap judgements about whether we'd like the other person as a friend, a workmate, a lover, and so on — all on the basis of what we see and hear, but mainly what we see. These first impressions last. We revise them when we learn more about the person, but only a little. Our overall view of someone is strongly coloured by those first five minutes.

What seems particularly unjust is that good-lookers are often credited with other plus points. Research has shown that when we are shown pictures of attractive people, we see them as having nicer personalities, as being more intelligent and talented, more friendly and outgoing, more sympathetic and responsive, and so on, than less attractive people. They are also held to be more likely to be successful — to hold top jobs, be more happily married, be better parents and have better lives generally — than unattractive people. But does attractiveness lead to success and happiness? Or does self-fulfilment lead to an aura which makes a person look attractive?

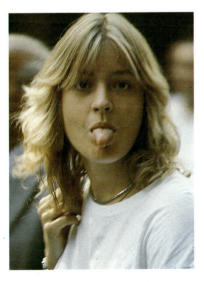

The face we're born with is entirely in the lap of the gods but, as George Orwell said, by the time we're fifty we all have the face we *deserve*. And here's where hope lies for all of us who don't look like Bo Derek or Richard Gere. Fortunately, people are more likely to notice the personality/ temperament/character written in a face than the facial features themselves. Social researchers have found that people generally agree about what counts as an ideal face in a photograph — for both sexes it would be clear wide eyes, a high forehead, even teeth, a straight nose and generally symmetrical features — but when was the last time you shook hands with a photograph? When we're face to face with people in the flesh, there's a lot more to it than symmetry.

Flashing your assets _____

Think of the most attractive person you know, and then think of the person who is best liked. Are they one and the same? If they are, try to decide whether it's the *qualities* they possess — their charm, sensitivity, sense of humour — that makes them seem attractive or if it's their *looks*. If they're two different people, how well do they conform to the image of perfection described above, and what is the extra something the popular friend has?

When it comes to real life friendships and not celluloid fantasies we care more about things like warmth, humour and honesty than we do about the circumference of a person's chest or the length of their eyelashes. Some of us may even find too much perfection daunting. The tall leggy blonde at the disco may be stunning to look at, but if she poses the threat of rejection to would-be partners she may find herself dancing less than the ordinary girl with the cheery smile.

If you think you're too imperfect a specimen to crawl out from under your stone, next time you're sitting on a bus count how many people are *really* perfect. Be ruthless! You're looking for flawless complexions, immaculate hair, oodles of style — the lot. Changing rooms are even better places to do your research. You'll find most of the human race is warty, bulgy and blemished — but lovable.

So how do you make the best of yourself? Here are a few tips.

■ **Start with what you've got.** If you're a generous size 14, you're not going to make a size 10 without a great deal of self denial and willpower, not to mention hunger pangs, but you can aim to be a beautiful size 14. We tend to have fixed ideas in our heads that as soon as we've grown our hair/lost weight/grown a beard we'll be ready to face the world, and hide ourselves away until the time is right. But the difference that a couple of inches on or off your waistline/shoulders/hips/biceps is going to make is marginal. You'd be better off using the time wasted hiding yourself developing a new interest or a new friendship.

■ **Ignore the flaws.** Forget your weak points and play up your stronger ones. We're often far too preoccupied with minor imperfections and go to elaborate and unnecessary lengths to hide them. People with crooked teeth, often keep their mouths shut; but what other people notice is an unsmiling face, not the odd tooth out of line.

■ **Use your face.** If it's your fortune, let it earn for you! You can have very irregular features and yet be considered attractive if your face is animated, if it's expressive and lively. Use those muscles to give beaming smiles and interested and interesting expressions. People can't respond to stiff faces.

■ **Smile.** Not an inane grin or a fixed jaw-grimace, but a smile of genuinely wide and generous proportions. Obviously not when people don't deserve it or when the situation doesn't warrant it, but try to give others the benefit of the doubt. People tolerate a lot if you smile at them.

■ **Dress up.** Our bodies may affect what people think of us but so does the way we cover them. Clothes do more than keep us warm and stop us getting arrested. They tell people how we see ourselves and how we want to be seen. So don't just copy styles you see on others. Innovate. Cut out a series of looks from your favourite magazines, then mix and match them to your style by superimposing them on a photograph of yourself.

■ **Cultivate your charm.** Perhaps the most important of all. Not a shallow, superficial charm that can be switched on and off at will, but one which comes from a positive approach to people, a genuine interest in them and an enthusiasm for what they have to tell you, so that you radiate good feelings about them and they can bask in those feelings.

■ **If other people frighten you,** you just might be doing the same to them! Concentrate on putting people at ease; it'll take your mind off what they're thinking of you.

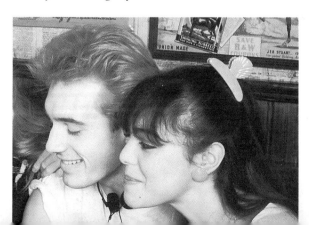

SHE'S FLASHING ONE OF HER MAJOR ASSETS — A SMILE THAT'S OPEN AND FRIENDLY.

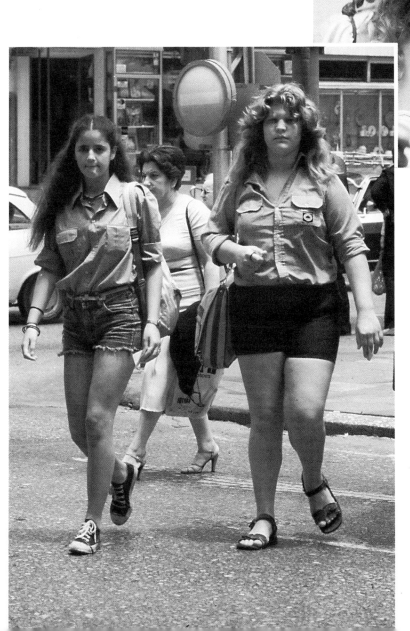

PEOPLE COME IN DIFFERENT SHAPES AND SIZES — SO MAKE THE BEST OF WHAT YOU'VE GOT.

13

You and your image

Much of the language we use to describe the way we present ourselves is borrowed from the theatre. We talk about putting on a good *performance*, getting our *act* together, playing a *part*. Even the word 'person' comes from the Greek word for a mask. So the words we use acknowledge the fact that all of us are always and everywhere playing a role.

This is probably never so true as when you're young and single. As you get older, you find someone else is doing the casting. As wife, husband, parent or boss, certain patterns of behaviour and lifestyle are going to be expected of you; people will expect you to behave in an appropriate way. At the same time, people are going to take a less lenient view of bizarre or outlandish behaviour. Flamboyant self-expression which passes for youthful colour gets labelled ostentatious as you get older; with the passage of time originality turns into eccentricity.

Right now you have the freedom to explore different looks and lifestyles without too much disapproval. Make the most of it. Treat this time of your life as a dress rehearsal. If you make mistakes they're not permanent.

There are a host of different parts you can choose from. Some are ready-made — you can be 'preppy' or 'punk', a Young Fogey or a New Romantic, an Urban Guerrilla or a Sloane Ranger, a Yuppy or a Yumpy … though of course by the time you read this some of these fashions will be defunct and have been replaced by others. These roles are there for the taking. All you need are the 'props' that go with them — the right clothes, language, music.

Why do people adopt fashions like these? Because most of us need to feel we belong to a particular group, and because extreme styles very clearly set us apart from the rest, show we're unique. They also bring us together with people we want to identify with. Being different from people who don't matter is actually being the same as people who do matter. It's as important to seem different from outsiders as it is to be the same as the in-crowd. Your image is a badge which says ' I belong with this group and we're different from the rest of you'.

What you've got to decide is how far you want to take an image on board wholesale and how far you want to make one for yourself. When you adopt an off-the-peg image, there's always the danger that you'll lose your own identity. Try to hang onto it. Decide what your own distinctive features are — style, behaviour, looks, personality — and make sure they're well served by, and shine through, the image you opt for. After all, you want to stand out from your set. Adopting an image without adapting it to *you* is just another way of conforming. The real challenge is to develop a style all of your own, a style you'll develop through life.

WE CAN'T CHANGE OUR FEATURES — BUT WE CAN USE THEM TO EXPRESS OUR PERSONALITY … AND THE RESULTS WILL CERTAINLY GET YOU NOTICED!

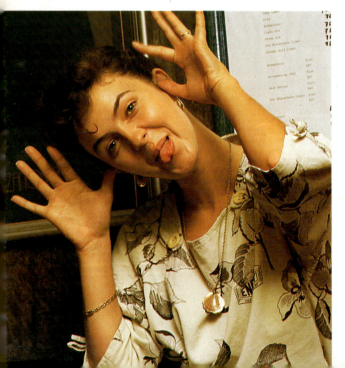
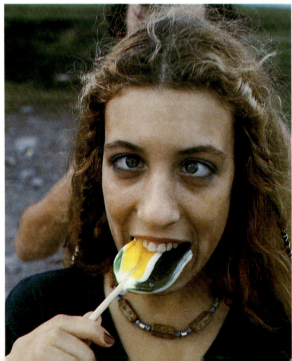

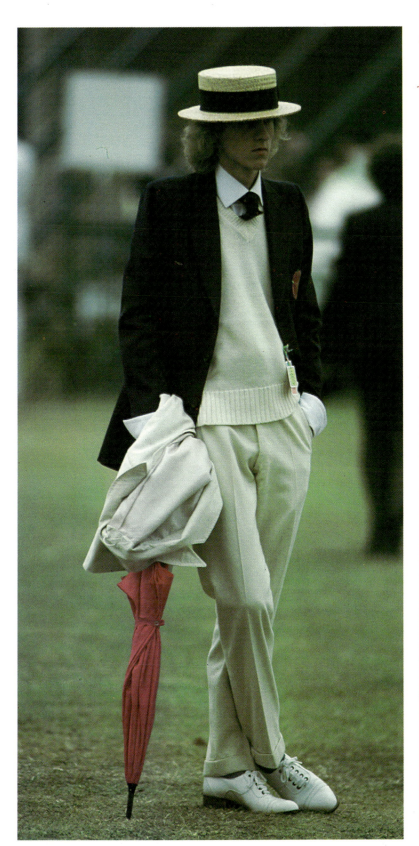

CHOOSE YOUR OWN IMAGE . . .

. . . THERE'S NO SHORTAGE OF OPTIONS.

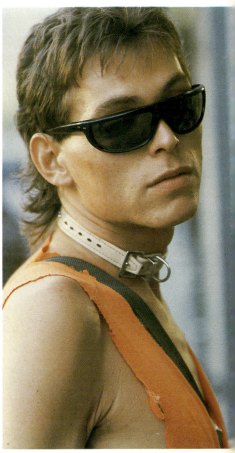

The real you

The face we present to the world is rarely our real face, or rather it is one of many. We wear different masks for different people and different situations — we have our party face, our interview face, our family face. We talk about 'putting on a brave face', about 'facing up to things', about someone being 'two-faced' when two of their faces don't match up. Like chameleons, we're all capable of blending in with our backgrounds.

You could argue that this is dishonest or insincere. But that would be a bit harsh. A little play-acting may be necessary to help life run smoothly. Imagine what it would be like if your feelings really were written on your face, if people could read your innermost thoughts, sense your fears and your emotions. There'd be a lot of flak flying around and a lot of bruised and battered egos. We'd all need hides like rhinoceroses. We're all capable of thinking ugly or wounding thoughts from time to time. It wouldn't do to have them on public display.

So we tend to edit our thoughts and censor our feelings for public consumption. We wear a mask that reveals the parts of us that will be accepted socially and conceals those that won't. This masking process goes beyond our faces. We mask with our whole bodies. We hold our heads upright along with our thoughts, and we hold our stomachs in along with our emotions. That way we protect our own feelings and avoid hurting those of others.

There are limits though to the extent to which we should 'keep up appearances'. To do so all the time would be a strain emotionally; sometimes we have to let the mask slip. It's important to know when and where to end the performance, finish the script, start being spontaneous. The danger is that if we don't, the mask becomes the only identity we have. When we say we 'can't get through' to someone we mean that we can't get past the mask to the real person underneath. So, does your image hide the real you?

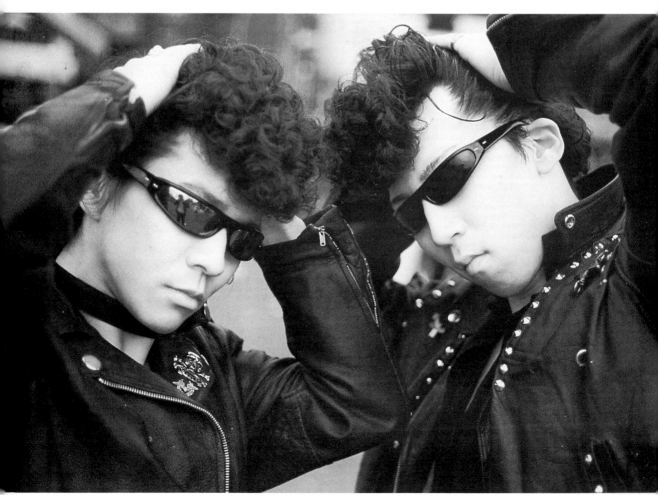

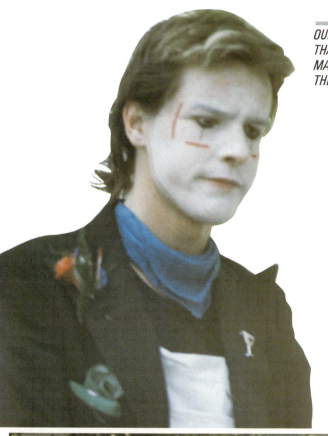

OUR CLOTHES HELP US TO IDENTIFY WITH OTHERS — AND THAT'S IMPORTANT. BUT IT'S JUST AS IMPORTANT TO MAKE SURE WE DON'T LOSE OUR OWN INDIVIDUALITY AT THE SAME TIME.

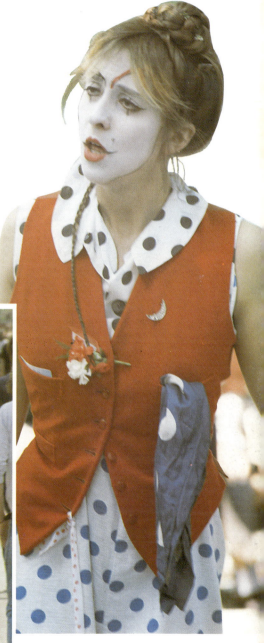

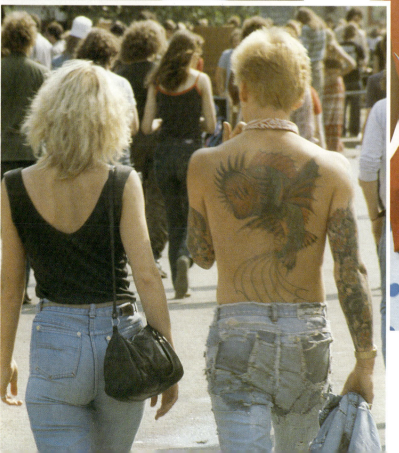

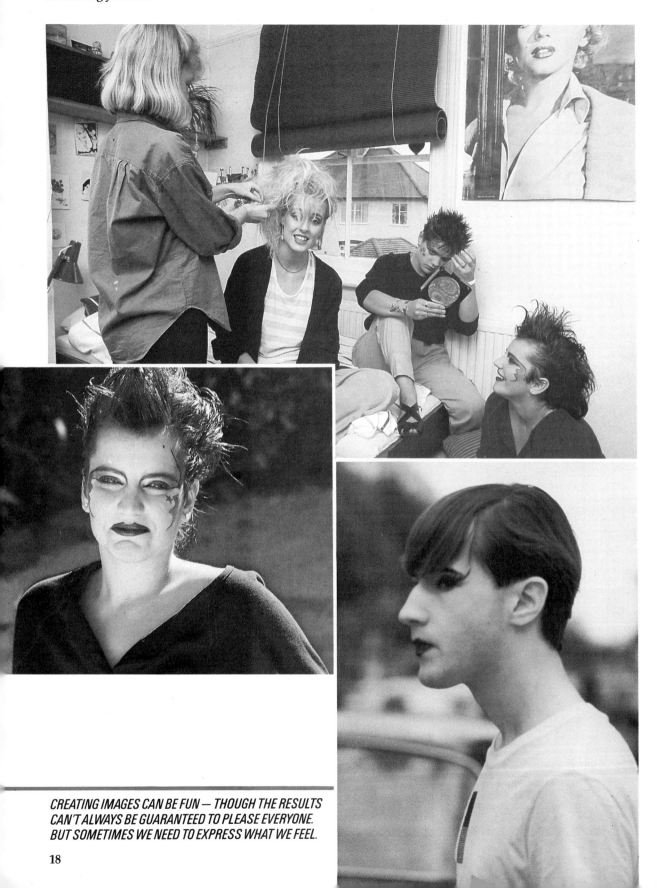

CREATING IMAGES CAN BE FUN — THOUGH THE RESULTS
CAN'T ALWAYS BE GUARANTEED TO PLEASE EVERYONE.
BUT SOMETIMES WE NEED TO EXPRESS WHAT WE FEEL.

■ **Don't wear an image like a mask.** People want to know *you*, not your mask. An image should flatter, not disguise. If you're aiming for the perfect cover-up, ask yourself what it is you're hiding and why you don't like it.

■ **Don't try to be someone else.** You won't make half such a good job of it! And he or she may want to look like you anyway!

■ **Aim for variation rather than transformation.** If you're given to overnight overhauls, ask yourself why you got so fed up with yesterday's image.

■ **Don't be afraid to be different.** You've nothing to lose but your anonymity. But make sure your style really expresses your personality. You'll be found out pretty quickly if it doesn't. Get a (really good!) friend to help you pin down what suits you best.

Unfortunately, the need to cover up their true selves is so deep-rooted in some people that they're unable to let down their defences even when they want to. They stick to safe, impersonal topics of conversation, like the price of audio tapes, and they don't get too close. Underneath they may be very vulnerable and sensitive, which makes them even more afraid to reveal their true feelings. They may have been in a close relationship where there was little chance of expressing the intimate side of themselves. Their family may have discouraged open displays of affection and feeling. From an early age most of us are taught — by parents, teachers, older people in general — to keep our emotions in check.

Fortunately no one ever succeeds in doing the job perfectly. We don't become automatons, programmed to respond at all times in socially acceptable ways. We may have control over some aspects of our behaviour, but by no means over all. Some things we have no control over, as you'll find out in the next chapter.

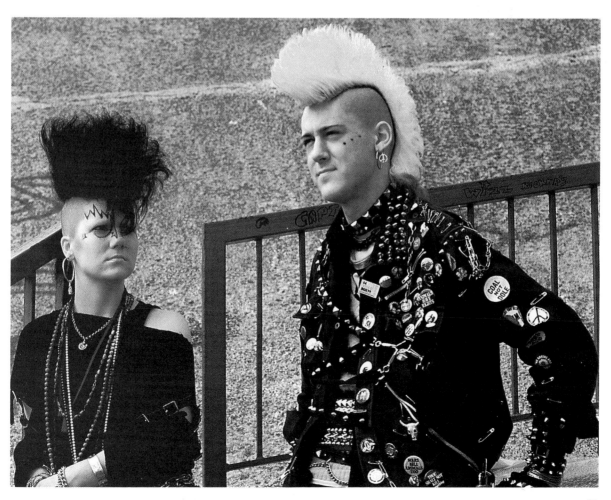

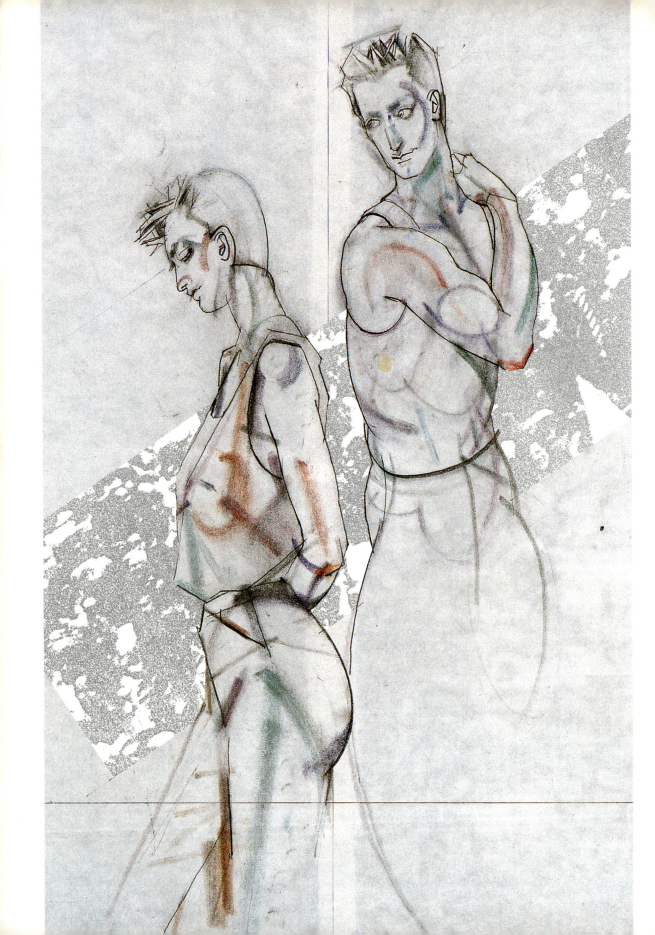

2
Body messages

All of us are capable of sending out signs and signals which speak volumes without our ever uttering a word. In fact, some social psychologists believe we do less than 10 per cent of our communicating through speech; the rest is done through a variety of 'non-verbal' signals. We lift an eyebrow in disbelief, we hunch our shoulders when we're tense, we wiggle our toes when we're excited. Often these gestures say things we find difficult to put into words. So, do our body messages hold the key to what we'd like to say but daren't?

Social psychologists used to think so. Decipher body language and look into the unspoken thoughts and intentions of your friends! Of course it's not that simple. It began with an American psychologist called Ray Birdwhistell in the late 1940s. He went to elaborate lengths to compile a vocabulary of nods, winks, taps and shrugs, and tried to translate them. A scratch of the nose, for example, signalled a lie or a disagreement; tightly folded arms indicated defensiveness and a need for self-protection. Body language was a code, and once the code was cracked we'd all be perfect communicators.

So much for the theory. In practice, there's always the possibility that someone is scratching their nose because it itches, or hugging herself because she's cold. A lot depends on the context and the person concerned. Crossed legs, bent legs, parallel legs, may well be clues to what a person is thinking, but they may just as well mean nothing at all. Again, we have to know something about the owner of the legs and the setting

The signals we send out are not always under our control. When we're sexually aroused, for example, the pupils of our eyes dilate automatically, our lips get fuller and redder and our complexion flushes. (When people apply lipstick and cheek blusher, or use black kohl to make their eyes look bigger, they're mimicking just these reactions.)

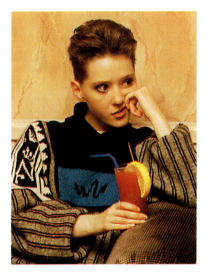

Understanding body language can be an aid to unscrambling mixed messages. Though the spoken word can convey extremely precise and truthful messages, we also use words to disguise the truth and sometimes our body movements give us away. If you keep your antennae sharp you may be able to pick up some of the meanings behind what people say. Coming shortly to this chapter is a quick hidden meanings course! The photos and their accompanying commentary are a guide only; once you're into the subject, you'll be able to pick up many other messages. You'll also become more aware of the impact of your own body language — the way you watch and listen to people, the way you touch and talk to them.

Close enough for comfort?

The simplest and most obvious type of body language is touch. The touch of a hand or an arm around someone's shoulders makes an instant bond between two people and is the most effective way possible of saying 'I like you'. Yet for many people, particularly in our society, it's also the most difficult. There's a kind of taboo on touching as a means of communication. We carry our bubbles of privacy around with us and we get offended if people burst them uninvited.

Yet there's plenty of evidence that we need body contact for our emotional growth. Babies thrive on being patted and stroked and cuddled. So do adults, but as we grow up we start receiving conflicting messages. Don't touch, we're told. Don't touch the goods on the counter, the food on our plates, ourselves even. It's not surprising that we eventually apply the 'don't touch' rule to people.

What happens is that touching gets tangled up with sex, so that 'don't touch' tends to mean 'don't touch sexually'. Cuddling or putting your arm around someone gets misinterpreted as a sexual advance. When we do touch, it's the sexually neutral parts of the body, like the shoulders, arms and head that we touch. Off-limits areas are those associated with sex — crotches, bottoms, hips, breasts.

Worse, especially for boys, is that touching is often associated with weakness and unmanliness. Men are far more likely than women to interpret a touch as a trigger for sexual intimacy, and far less likely to read it as a sign of warmth and affection. One of the sad results of this is that couples who have been together for some time (and even some who haven't) complain that they don't get cuddles any more. They've forgotten how to display closeness out of bed, how to display warmth and intimacy to each other outside of sex. Then when it comes to actually making love, even that is impoverished by their inability to express physical affection.

All this is a great shame. It's a mistake to assume that others will think less of us if we ditch our inhibitions and show some physical affection. None of us is taken in by a frosty peck on the cheek or an over-enthusiastic 'hail-fellow-well-met' backslap, but there's something very heart-warming about a big bear hug between two men who share a real bond of affection, or two girls companionably linking arms.

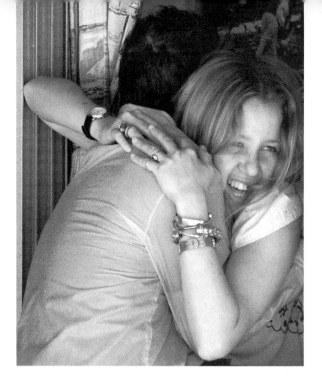

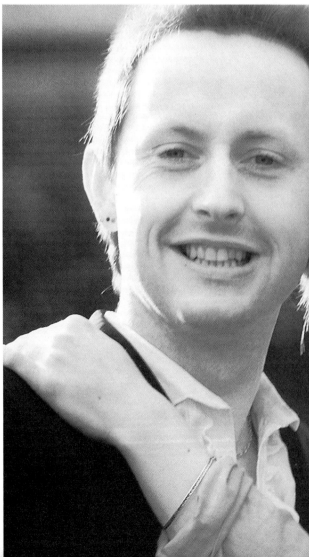

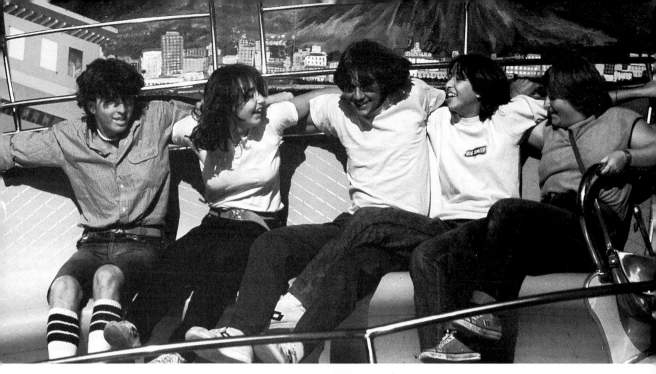

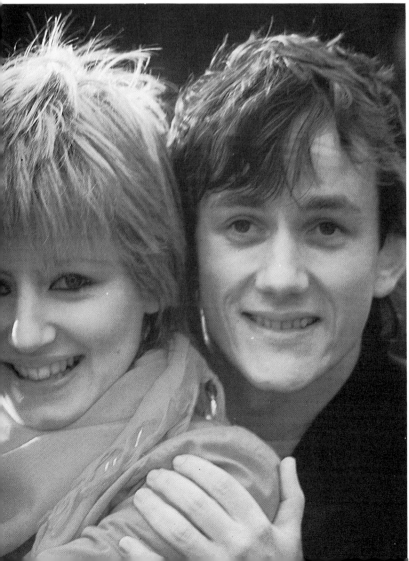

WE ALL NEED BODY CONTACT FOR
EMOTIONAL GROWTH, SO BURST THE
BUBBLE OF PRIVACY THAT
SURROUNDS YOU — AND HAVE SOME
FUN AT THE SAME TIME.

AN ARM LIGHTLY RESTING ON
SOMEONE'S KNEE...

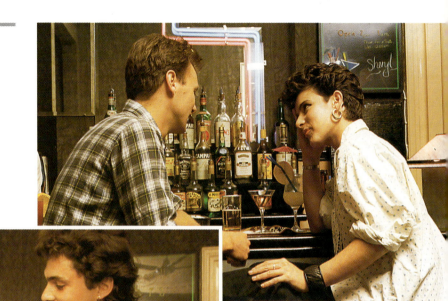

...A MOCK SCUFFLE...

...ARMS ROUND SHOULDERS AND
WAISTS...

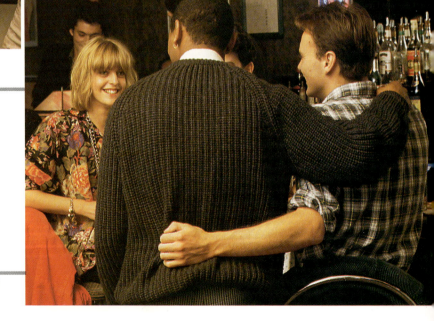

...ALL EFFECTIVE WAYS OF GETTING
ACROSS WARMTH AND AFFECTION.

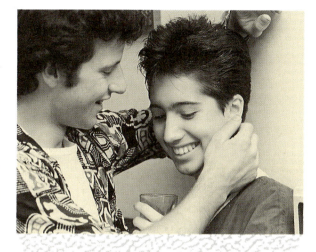

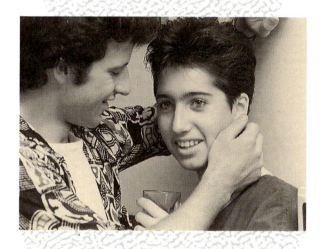

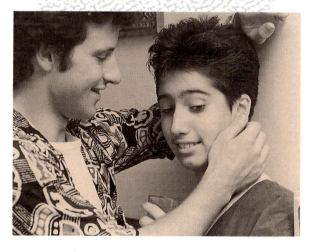

Eye power

When it comes to transmitting direct messages, the eyes have it. Our two ocular orbs are the most powerful communicators we have. Show the average male a picture of a naked female and his pupils become twice as large as normal and he can't do a thing about it. But there are ways in which we can control what our eyes say. It all depends on how we maintain eye contact and for how long.

In a sense the eyes are the only appropriate bit of another human being to look at. For one thing they're in roughly the same place and at the right height and level! Start looking down to someone's collar and you'll find they're picking non-existent hairs off it in no time.

Making direct eye contact is the natural way to engage someone's attention. Yet for some people it's also the most difficult. When they should be gazing meaningfully into someone's eyes, they're examining their fingernails or the cutlery. Too little eye contact suggests insincerity and shiftiness, even anger and resentment, but too much can be offensive. You've probably been told it's rude to stare, and so it is. We reserve an unblinking gaze for things other than people — for objects and animals. Staring at someone is equivalent to treating them as a non-person. Too much eye contact, then, signifies either a lack of respect or a wish to dominate or intimidate.

Clearly the secret lies in striking a balance. Sometimes we have no difficulty making eye contact when we're discussing impersonal or easy topics, but we tend to look away or only fleetingly meet the other person's eyes if we're talking about something intimate or difficult. As a general rule, it's probably better to err on the side of too much eye contact than too little. Your companion can always look away.

Because our eyes are a natural focus of attention, the whole area around them presents lots of possibilities for getting messages across, from a wink ('I know what you're thinking', 'It's not that serious') to a raising of eyebrows ('Is he kidding?', 'You're taking a bit of a risk!'). Don't neglect them. Learn to smile with your eyes as well as your mouth. Practise in front of the mirror — keep your mouth in a straight line and try to put a smile on your face! By bringing into play all the muscles in the eye area, you'll give a far more natural and effective smile than you will with your lips alone.

LEFT: HE'S TOO CLOSE FOR COMFORT SO NO MATTER HOW HARD HE TRIES, SHE'S AVOIDING ANY MEANINGFUL EYE CONTACT.

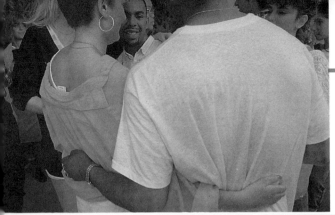

LEFT: TOUCHING MAKES AN INSTANT BOND. PUTTING YOUR ARM AROUND SOMEONE IS THE SIMPLEST AND EASIEST WAY OF SAYING YOU LIKE THEM.

BELOW: HANDS PROTECTIVELY CLASPED, HE DOESN'T SEEM TO NEED CONTACT. BUT HIS SIDELONG GLANCE TELLS US HE'D LIKE TO BE PART OF WHAT'S GOING ON IN THE GROUP.

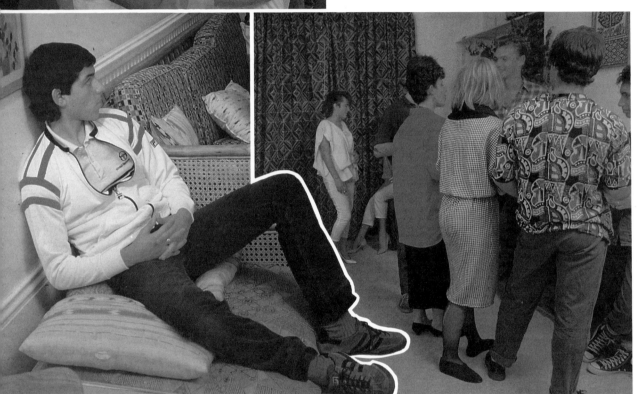

Melting and freezing _____

Obviously we can't go around stroking and hugging just anyone! That could lead to trouble. Freedom to touch varies from one individual to another and from one setting to another. Some of us are better than others at touching and being touched. Some people enjoy bodily contact and respond readily to it; others tend to freeze up and withdraw.

Freezing up is really a way of keeping things under control. People who freeze may have been taught that their quite normal need for affection is something to be ashamed of; or they may have quite normal sexual fantasies that they are afraid of revealing by letting the other person get too close. Rather than be rejected for being too open, they shy away from contact and, in effect, do the rejecting themselves. Control is achieved, but the price is loneliness.

Withdrawing from contact is one way of protecting a frail or low self-image. Underneath the person is actually saying 'I can't believe that I'm huggable/nice to be near'. But the fact that someone is making the effort to be near them should be telling them the opposite. Inside they long for contact, but they fear rebuff even more, and so they put up the barriers.

Then again, not every social setting calls for close contact. What would be appropriate conduct at a party wouldn't do for the office or among strangers in a public place. Psychologists have worked out a pattern of physical zones corresponding to social settings. As a rough and ready guide, direct touching is OK when you're on intimate terms, arm's length when you're being friendly and body length for more formal social encounters. You can often spot people negotiating their

RIGHT: CREATING SOCIAL DISTANCE: THE HAND ON HER CHEEK IS MAKING AN EFFECTIVE BARRIER BETWEEN THESE TWO. CROSSED LEGS AND A PROTECTIVE HAND COMPLETE THE DEFENCE.

BELOW: CLOSING SOCIAL DISTANCE: THEY'RE PAST THE SMALL TALK AND ANY MINUTE NOW SHE'LL BE DOWN FROM THAT PERCH AND WITHIN ARM'S REACH.

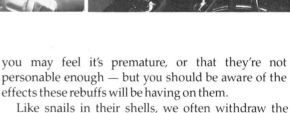

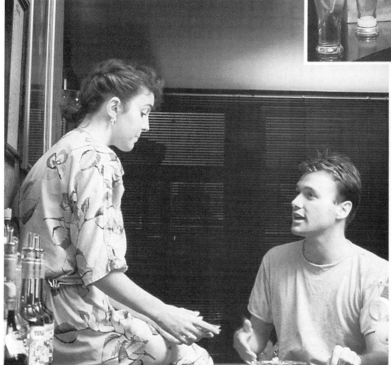

body space in this way, hopping backwards and forwards and skirting round each other as if they're on pogo sticks, trying to establish whether the 'intimacy' or 'social friends' distance feels right for them.

When we're forced closer than seems appropriate for the social setting we feel uncomfortable and we use a variety of ploys to create distance. Next time you're in a lift, or a crowded bus or train, watch how people stare past or through their neighbours, or slip a newspaper between others and themselves. If people take advantage of this sort of nearness, we understandably take exception (or the nearest sharp object) to them.

But by the same token, it's understandable if people take offence when the social setting says touch and you use space to distance yourself. There may be a genuine reason why you don't feel like accepting a gesture —

you may feel it's premature, or that they're not personable enough — but you should be aware of the effects these rebuffs will be having on them.

Like snails in their shells, we often withdraw the soft, vulnerable bits of ourselves and expose only a cold, hard, protective shell. But snails with their feelers withdrawn go nowhere fast! So in the spirit of 'nothing ventured, nothing gained', stretch out a little, gesture outwards. If you're not a natural toucher but feel you'd like more body contact, take small steps to begin with: a light touch on the arm to emphasize a point; playful gestures — walking your fingers up someone's arm, putting hands over eyes from behind, even throwing a mock punch — are good ice breakers; hooking an arm around a friend's neck or ruffling their hair (not if it's newly coiffed!).

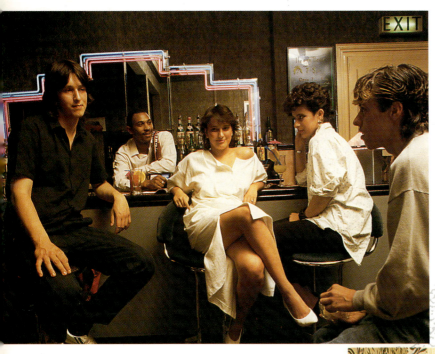

LEFT: COUNT THE COME-ONS HERE. A LOT OF NAKED FLESH IS ESCAPING FROM THAT DRESS, THE POSTURE IS COMPLETELY OPEN AND THE SMILE IS COME-HITHER.

BELOW: HE'S TELLING THE TRUTH WITH HIS WHOLE BODY: PALMS AND CHIN UP, GAZE DIRECT, AND LEG PLANTED FIRMLY FORWARD CHALLENGING ANYONE TO DOUBT HIS HONESTY.

BELOW: THERE'S A MIXED MESSAGE HERE. SITTING ON A TABLE, ONE OF THE GROUP HAS RAISED HIS HEIGHT, AND THEREFORE HIS SOCIAL POSITION, HANDS SPREAD FIRMLY IN COMPLETE CONTROL. BUT THERE'S A GIVE AWAY. IF HE WAS REALLY AT EASE HIS ANKLES WOULD BE RELAXED. AS IT IS, HIS FEET ARE RIGIDLY AT RIGHT-ANGLES TO HIS LEGS.

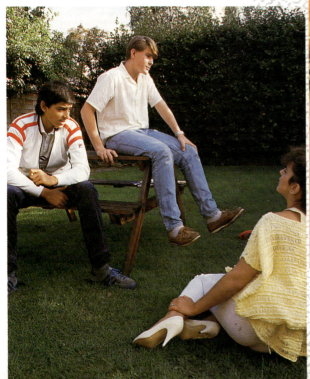

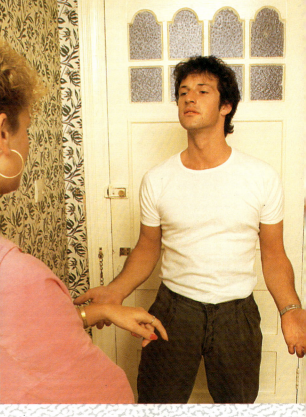

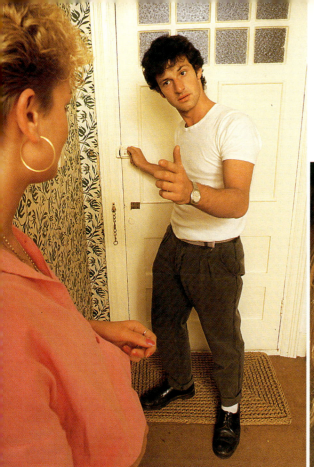

LEFT: PARTING SHOT — NOTICE HIS HAND ON THE DOORKNOB, WHAT HE'S SAYING IS PROBABLY DIFFICULT AND MAYBE A LITTLE PAINFUL, AND THAT HAND IS POISED TO ALLOW A QUICK GET AWAY AND ALSO TO SAY THAT THIS IS HIS FINAL WORD.

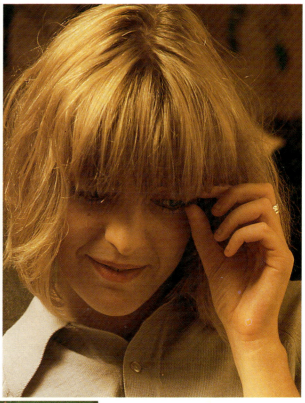

ABOVE: SHE HASN'T REALLY GOT AN EYELASH IN HER EYE BUT IT'S A GOOD WAY OF HIDING HALF HER FACE, WHICH IS SET TO BETRAY A TURMOIL OF FEELINGS.

LEFT: NO POINT IN TRYING TO GET IN ON THIS ACT! THEY'RE A SELF-CONTAINED GROUP WITH CLOSED MEMBERSHIP AND TO SHOW THIS THEY'VE CO-ORDINATED THEIR KNEES AND THEIR ELBOWS TO FORM A CLOSED CIRCLE.

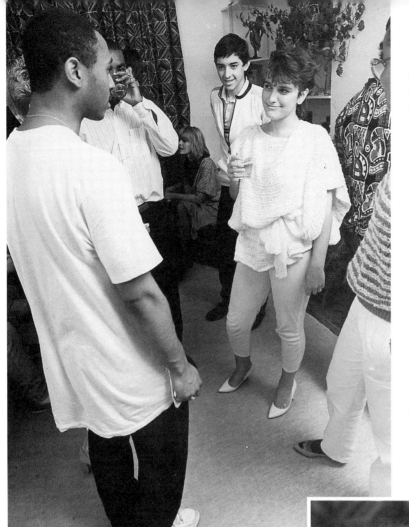

LEFT: A PROMISING ENCOUNTER. HIS ARMS ARE LOOSE BY HIS SIDE, BODY HELD FORWARD, INDICATING A WILLINGNESS TO MAKE FRIENDS. FOR HER PART, HER HEAD IS TILTED TOWARDS ONE SIDE, SHOWING SHE'S CURIOUS AND INTERESTED.

BELOW: LISTENING IS NOT A PASSIVE ACTIVITY. HIS ATTENTIVE FACIAL EXPRESSION, HEAD ON ONE SIDE, TELLS HER THAT HE'S INTERESTED IN WHAT SHE'S SAYING.

BELOW: HE'S BITING THE NAIL ON HIS LITTLE FINGER WITH A PENSIVE LOOK. IT WOULDN'T DO FOR A COOL CHARACTER LIKE HIM TO BE SEEN TO BE SUCKING HIS THUMB, BUT THAT'S THE EXACT EQUIVALENT OF WHAT HE'S DOING. IT SHOWS HE'S NOT AS SECURE OR CONFIDENT AS HE'D LIKE TO SUGGEST.

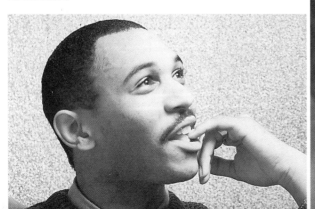

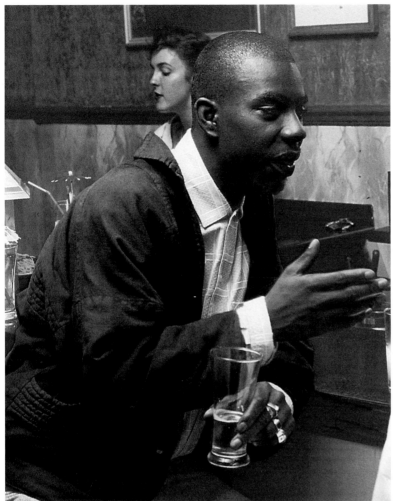

LEFT: HE'S USING HIS OUTSTRETCHED HAND TO CONFIRM AND DRIVE HOME HIS MESSAGE. IT'S DIRECT, TO THE POINT, AND HE MEANS IT.

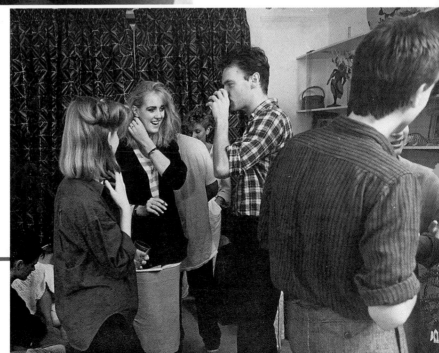

RIGHT: SOME EXPERTS BELIEVE THAT HAIR-TOUCHING IS A SIGN OF SEXUAL INTEREST. I WONDER IF HE'S AWARE OF THE IMPRESSION HE'S CREATING?

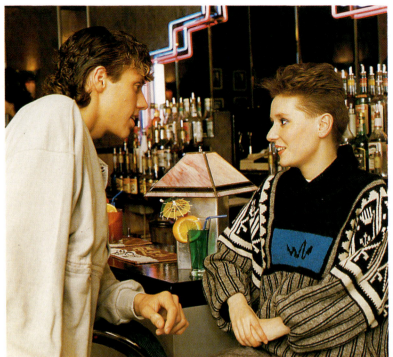

LEFT: YOU CAN FEEL THE TENSION AND FEAR IN THE HUNCHED SHOULDERS AND TIGHTLY CLASPED HANDS. IF HE'S GOING TO MAKE ANY HEADWAY WITH HER, HE'S GOING TO HAVE TO MAKE A LOT OF REASSURING NOISES FIRST.

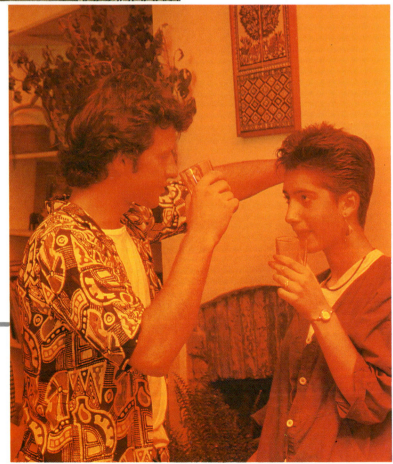

RIGHT: A TYPICAL PARTY STANCE. SHE'S USING THE WALL FOR SUPPORT AND SECURITY AND IS NONE TOO SURE OF HERSELF. HE'D LIKE TO BE A BIT MORE SURE OF HER AND SO IS STAKING HIS CLAIM ON HER WITH OUTSTRETCHED ARM — MAKING A GET-AWAY POSSIBLE ONLY ON ONE FRONT.

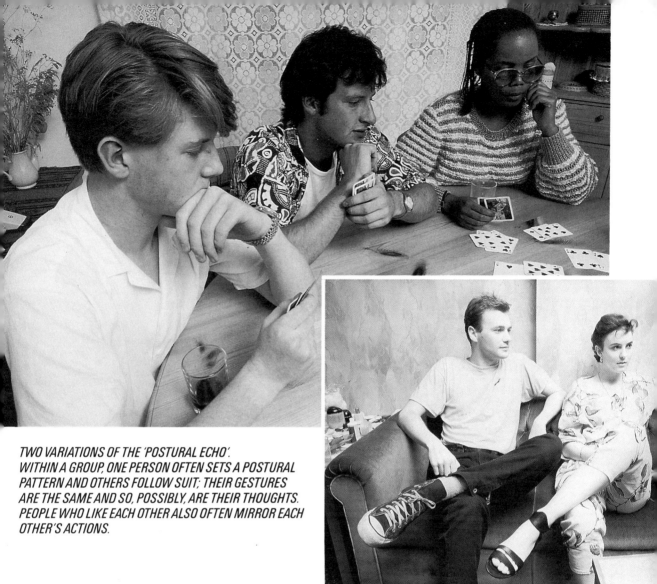

TWO VARIATIONS OF THE 'POSTURAL ECHO'.
WITHIN A GROUP, ONE PERSON OFTEN SETS A POSTURAL
PATTERN AND OTHERS FOLLOW SUIT; THEIR GESTURES
ARE THE SAME AND SO, POSSIBLY, ARE THEIR THOUGHTS.
PEOPLE WHO LIKE EACH OTHER ALSO OFTEN MIRROR EACH
OTHER'S ACTIONS.

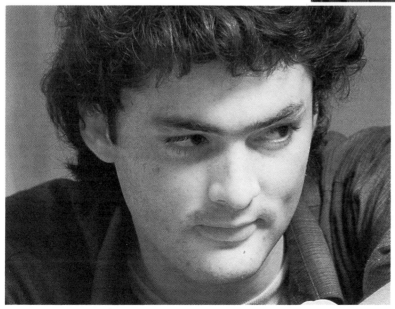

LEFT: THIS WICKED LOOK SAYS 'MY
INTENTIONS TOWARDS YOU ARE NOT
ENTIRELY HONOURABLE, BUT I DON'T
BELIEVE YOURS ARE EITHER, SO WHAT
ARE WE WAITING FOR?'

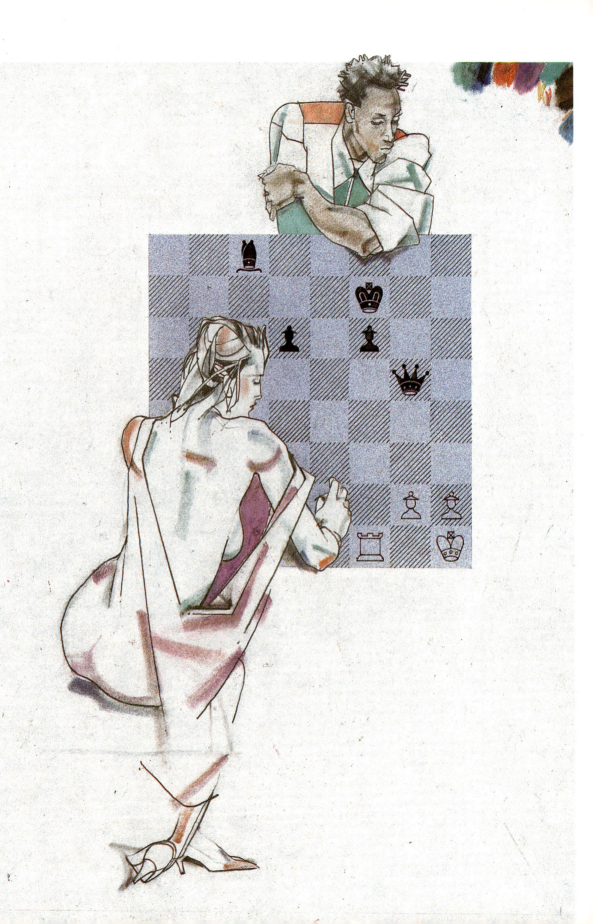

3 Meeting up and making out

Friendship is a blanket term we apply to all sorts of relationships, from those between members of a football team to very close one-to-one relationships. And 'being friendly' can describe anything from helping an old lady across the road to lending a sympathetic ear to the most intimate problems of a very special friend. All of us need to experience the full range of types of friendship. We need to feel the sense of belonging, of comradeship, that comes from being part of a gang, group, club or community. And we also need the closer, more intimate bond that develops between special personal friends.

In our open kind of society, it's fairly easy to make casual friendships. We constantly meet new sets of people to draw friends from. We enter new groups and make new acquaintances without mourning too much the loss of the old ones. Yet *real* friends, the bare-your-soul variety, are more difficult to come by.

These kind of friends are vital, whether they are of the same or the opposite sex. They're a reliable source of support and pleasure. So when you do make close friends, put a high priority on keeping them. Don't neglect them. Give them time and treat them well. Show them affection and genuine interest, and accept them as they are. Really close friendships need to be worked at, nurtured, treasured. Cultivated carefully, they can last a lifetime.

Where do you meet people?

It's not difficult to meet 'people', but it can be difficult to meet people you'll like and have something in common with. That's why there are so many commercially-run organizations that promise to match like with like.

Where you meet people is important because it acts as a kind of weeding out process. You're unlikely to meet war games enthusiasts on a civil rights march, or good drinking companions at a teetotallers' convention! It's a good idea to meet people in a variety of settings, not just the familiar stamping grounds of mate-seekers, like parties and discos. You *may* meet someone you like at a disco, having blown a week's pay on a stunning new outfit, but your chances of meeting someone in the local supermarket, library or sports club are just as great. You're going to need friends as well as lovers, and *doing* things together, sharing an interest, is a better basis for friendship than just spending time together. If the friendship turns out to be non-platonic, that's a bonus.

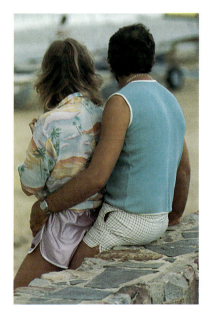

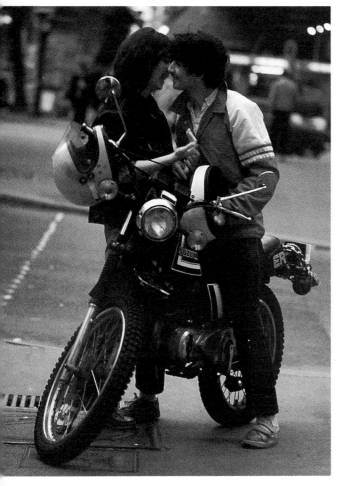

YOU WON'T ALWAYS MEET UP IN A ROMANTIC SETTING LOOKING YOUR GLAMOROUS BEST...

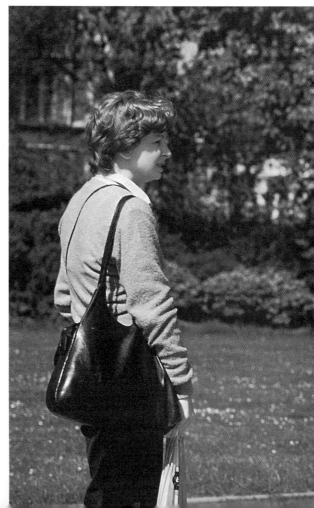

The other advantage of meeting people in everyday settings is that we form more realistic impressions of each other when we're not decked out in our glad rags and greasepaint, perfumed and aftershaved. This makes for more genuine and honest relationships. If you meet someone when you're already looking your best, you're going to have a lot to live up to. But imagine the effect, if you first met that person as your normal unadorned self, of really dressing up!

So don't dismiss everyday encounters in your search for friends, romantic or otherwise. Ordinary can lead to extraordinary. Here are some of the replies we got when we asked a number of people how they'd met the person they described as their best friend (same or opposite sex).

> 'He's a policeman and our house was on his beat. We used to hang out of the upstairs window and poke fun at him.' LENA

> 'We met at a university sit-in; we were sitting-in near each other and got chatting.' SUE

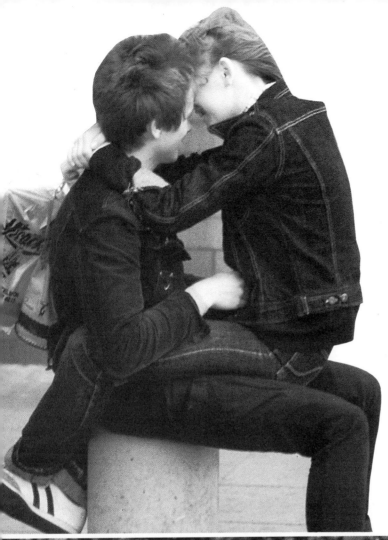

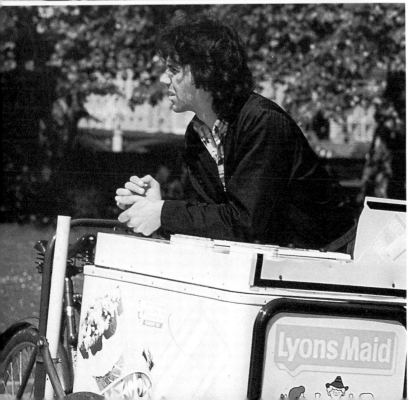

... EVERYDAY ENCOUNTERS TAKE PLACE IN EVERYDAY PLACES.

'She was working in the next office to me. We used to pull faces at each other through the glass, that sort of thing. We got together at the Christmas party.' PETER

'It was my first job and we both worked in the mailroom. He got up my nose because he wrote poetry while I did all the work. I got really mad at him.' GAIL

'We go to work on the same train every day. One day on the way home I said to him "I shouldn't sit there, I've got some really smelly cheese in my bag". Fortunately for me he didn't mind the cheese.' DENISE

'We met at a party... a friend's twenty-first.' TONY

'We met in a pub. I'd never seen her before. My mate chatted her and her friend up. Nothing to do with me, honest!' MARTIN

'The chain came off my bicycle — it has a habit of doing that whenever I forget to change down from second to first. Suddenly he zoomed around the corner in his old banger, saw me struggling to put the chain back on and gave me a whiter than white towel to wipe my hands on! We got talking, then we went for a drink...' ANNE

Notice how few of these first encounters fit into the typical dating scenario. And notice how many of them have a work theme, which is hardly surprising. We spend a lot of time at work, we're forced into close proximity with colleagues, and we often share achievements and problems which bring us even closer. If people can put up with you when your nerves are in ribbons and you're tetchy and tired at the end of the day, they can put up with you any time! Friendships made at work stand a good chance of lasting.

Joining classes and interest groups is another way of making friends. Even in these days of disappearing sexual stereotypes there is a degree of segregation of the sexes in terms of interests. No prizes for guessing which sex predominates (a) in pottery and dressmaking and (b) in car maintenance and carpentry. So a wily choice of class/interest group might include the sex selection factor! Obviously, you should like what you're doing or you won't stay the course long enough to make friends. However, not everyone is working. If you're looking for a job, or having a deliberate break from the routine, voluntary groups are a good source of like-minded people.

BEFORE YOU CAN MAKE OUT YOU HAVE TO MEET UP. GETTING OUT AND ABOUT INCREASES YOUR CHANCES OF FINDING NEW FRIENDS AND POTENTIAL LOVERS.

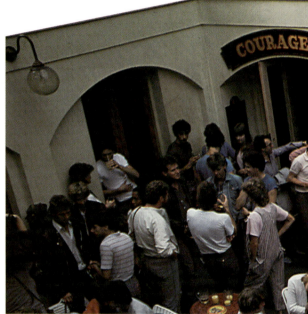

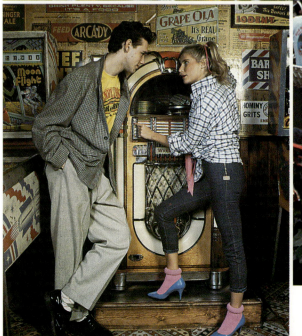

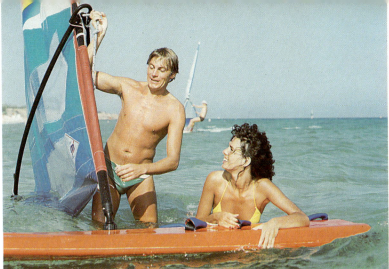

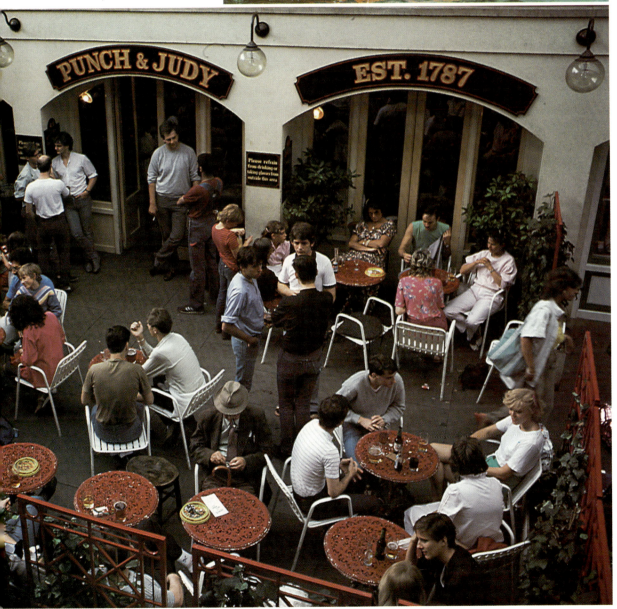

The agency solution

If you're feeling lonely — if you've just left home, for example, or if you've just broken up with someone — don't be too proud to use friendship agencies. Many of these provide a very useful service. It's simply not true that they serve the needs of the 'runners-up' rather than the 'favourites' in life. The idea of meeting up through singles clubs, computer dating agencies or the small ads is no more odd than going along to a dance and expecting to meet a soulmate. In fact going to a dance may be much more of a gamble. At least in the case of friendship clubs and computer dating agencies some effort is likely to have gone into finding you a match. You may get a few crackpots and weirdos, but the spread is about the same as you'll find anywhere else.

What you're less likely to get from these organizations is a ready-made feeling of togetherness. When you go to someone's party, you're likely to have something in common with the other guests simply by virtue of knowing your host and having been invited. If you set out to find friends in places where there's likely to be a very wide cross-section of people, where no pre-selecting has been done for you, you may have to put more effort into sorting out what is wheat and what is chaff for you personally.

One thing worth remembering about singles clubs is that quite a high proportion of members will have recently ended a long-term relationship and still be working through the painful after-effects. If you're the type who finds other people's problems a challenge, this won't bother you. But if you don't enjoy being a shoulder to weep on, think again.

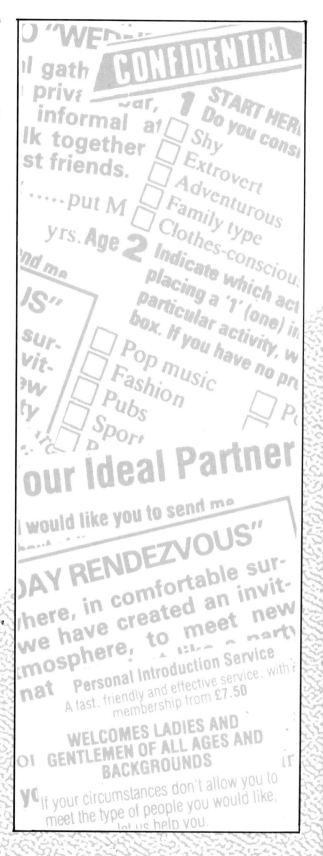

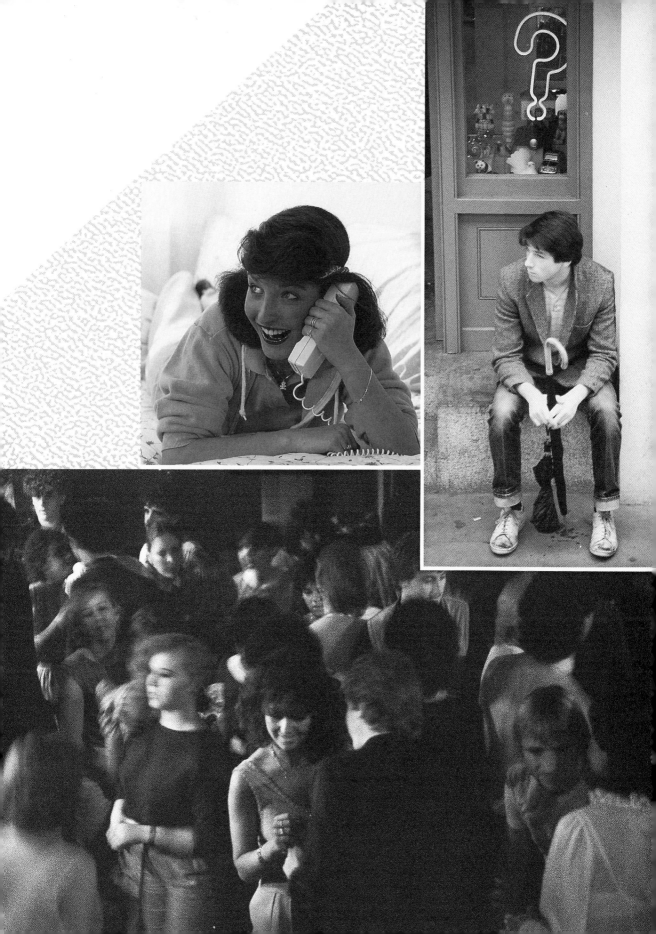

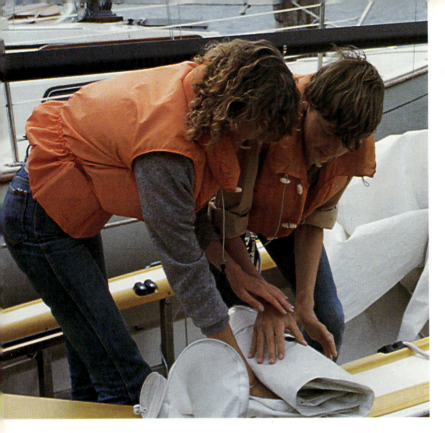

IT TAKES TWO TO MAKE A SUCCESSFUL PARTNERSHIP; WHO GOES FIRST DOESN'T REALLY MATTER — AS LONG AS IT ALL GOES WELL

Making overtures

Who makes the first move? Who takes the sexual initiative? By convention it's usually the man. He's the one who is expected to do the phoning and inviting, foot the bill, and take the lead generally. Many men are taught, by upbringing or tradition, that manliness depends on taking the initiative with women. In the same way, women traditionally have *not* been expected to make the first move — not in dating, dancing or in bed — but to wait passively for male overtures to be made.

In practice, of course, all this is an illusion. In their own discreet fashion women often make it quite clear that they have designs on a man. They signal interest by dropping hints, dressing up, giving the glad eye, and making themselves available. If they're too forward they're afraid they will be thought easy, or be laughed at, or worst of all rejected. But don't men feel that way too? Do we really need to go through these charades?

There's no basis in biology for this 'he chases, she runs' sort of behaviour. Animals go dutch when it comes to dating, or even reverse the roles. Look at the way peacocks strut around giving the come-on to the hens. And in feline affairs the female is only sexually available for a few days at a time so she doesn't sit around waiting for an interested tom to wander by. Nor is the male initiative common to all human societies. Among the Gaves, in India, the girl asks for the boy's hand in marriage and he's carried off by force and in tears from his weeping parents.

Many men and women manage to function as equals in the workplace or among friends, but revert to the old familiar patterns in the sexual arena. Many women feel uncomfortable and insecure about making the first move. And for every man who can truthfully say he would welcome more female initiative, there's another who is paralysed by the thought. Consider these two reactions:

'I liked the idea. I liked the thought of going out with someone who felt good about herself, confident enough to ring me. It was great. All I had to do was sit by the phone and this nice, attractive girl asked me out. Absolutely no hang-ups at all. She put the make on me — it made a nice change. I wish more would do it!' ED

'I'd run a mile! Well, I wouldn't, I'd let her down gently. I wouldn't want to hurt her feelings because it would take some courage. But I'd probably think, first off, that she had to be a bit hard up, not to choose me, I mean, just to have to ring anybody. Maybe I'm old-fashioned, but I can't see anything wrong with keeping things as they are.' DON

The first comment, notice, is based on experience;

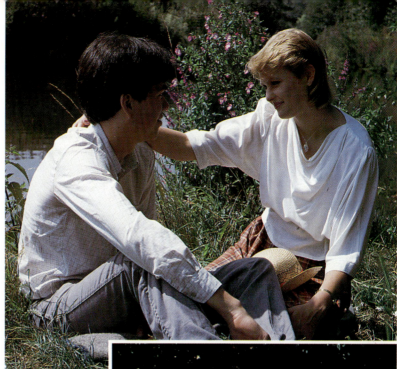

the second is not. Fairness alone dictates that women should take the initiative. The fact is that the 'man-as-active-predator' and 'woman-as-passive-prey' divide suits no one. Men have to bear the full brunt of rejection and are denied the flattery of women's sexual advances; women are left with the unpleasant business of fending men off and feeling frustrated at not being able to make their sexual interest clear.

Chatting someone up (see page 50) often takes a good deal of courage and men are not always brave nor women always timid. Research shows that women, when the time and place are right, are every bit as capable as men of taking the initiative. One study at a male strip show demonstrated that women are easily a match for men when it comes to cat-calling, stomping and yelling; they also took pleasure in propositioning the stripper.

Who takes the sexual initiative, then, has more to do with our risk-taking tendencies than the fact of being male or female. It's actually more useful to regard a willingness to take chances as a personality trait rather than a sex-related trait. Just think, there are probably scores of beautifully compatible couples in the world who never managed to get together simply because they stayed glued to the old sexual stereotypes!

So how do you rate as a risk-taker? And how does the special person in your life rate? Which of you made the first move?

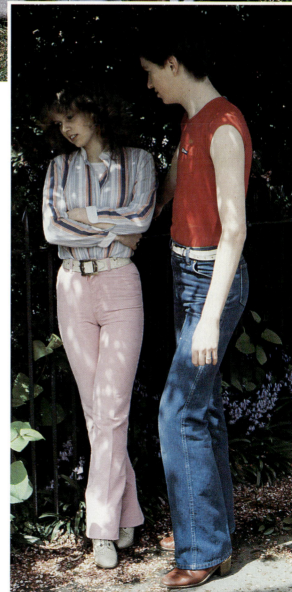

What are your risk-taking tendencies?

The statements below describe very different attitudes to dealing with people, money and health. Look at those on the right-hand side of the list and those on the left; and then decide which is the closest to the way you'd talk about yourself. If you seem to fall between the two extremes, put a ring round (5). Otherwise, put a ring round the number you feel best represents how strongly you feel on the issue. For example, in the first statement, if wild horses would *never* get you speaking on a public platform, circle (9), if you might be persuaded after a drop of Dutch courage, circle (6), and if you wouldn't turn a hair at the thought, circle (1) or (2). Add up the numbers you've circled.

STATEMENT		STATEMENT
I hate speaking or having to appear in public	1 2 3 4 5 6 7 8 9	I get a definite buzz out of performing in front of people
Generally speaking, I prefer to dress and make up conservatively	1 2 3 4 5 6 7 8 9	The more outlandish fashions in makeup and dress appeal to me personally
The most important factors in a job, for me, are security and a steady income	1 2 3 4 5 6 7 8 9	If a job looked exciting enough, I'd take a chance on it paying well
At parties, I tend to wait for someone to speak to me rather than make the first move	1 2 3 4 5 6 7 8 9	I'm quite happy to just bowl up to someone and strike up a conversation at a party
I feel more comfortable going with the crowd, than branching out on my own	1 2 3 4 5 6 7 8 9	I prefer to step out of line and be different, rather than to appear too conformist
If I couldn't find a road I was looking for I'd look in a street-finder rather than ask someone	1 2 3 4 5 6 7 8 9	If I'd lost my way, the first thing I'd do would be to ask someone
The thought of hang-gliding fills me with horror	1 2 3 4 5 6 7 8 9	If I had the chance to go hang-gliding, I'd take it
I'd never go out without checking that all the doors are locked	1 2 3 4 5 6 7 8 9	I have, on occasion, popped out leaving a door unlocked
I've never filled in football pools, played on fruit machines, or gambled in any way	1 2 3 4 5 6 7 8 9	I quite often take part in some form of gambling
I would never go into a restaurant or to the cinema on my own. I'd rather stay at home	1 2 3 4 5 6 7 8 9	If I wanted to have a meal or see a film, I wouldn't hesitate to go on my own. You never know who you might meet!

Your score

If you've scored *under* **25** then you're the sort who will avoid taking risks at all costs. You prefer the predictable humdrum of everyday life. You cut your losses to a minimum but adopting this strategy won't bring you any major gains in life either. If you've scored between **25** and **50**, you're the type who prefers life to be not too traumatic, but if the rewards seem worth having, you'll stick your neck out a little.

With a score of over **50** but under **75**, then you're a firm believer in the maxim 'Nothing ventured, nothing gained'. You're prepared to put yourself on the line, take a few chances, but with just enough caution to give you some self-protection. A score of **75** or over? You're a born gambler. Your life is likely to be littered with broken hearts, bones and banks, but no-one could ever say it was boring!

TAKE MORE CHANCES...

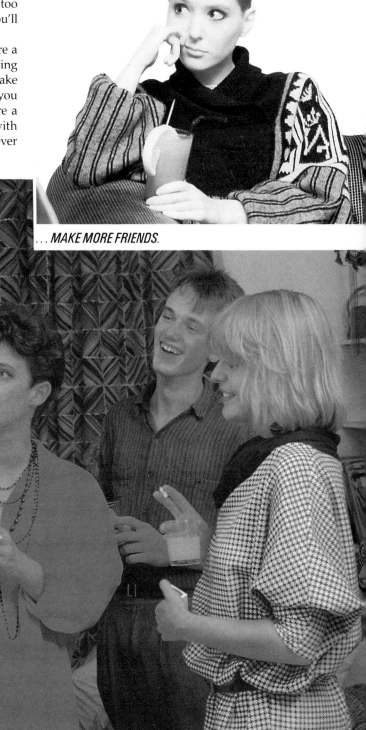

...MAKE MORE FRIENDS.

Feeling lonely

Everyone feels lonely at times. The phone doesn't ring, no one drops by and you feel there's not a soul out there who would really care if you suddenly disappeared off the face of the earth. Sometimes of course we feel lonely even when we're surrounded by people, or when we're with someone we love.

The need for companionship is as keen as the need for food and drink. There's nothing as depressing as having no one to share your thoughts and feelings with. But there's a big difference between feeling lonely and being on your own. They're far from being the same thing. A lot depends on whether you are on your own by choice. If you have friends you can contact if you want to, then settling for an evening at home may be more of a luxury than an ordeal.

Many people try to fend off feelings of loneliness by cramming their lives chock-full of social activities which don't necessarily solve the problem, or only temporarily. Companionship has more to do with quality than quantity. It's not so much a matter of collecting acquaintances and filling your diary as finding one or two really good friends you can turn to, confide in, trust, and enjoy being with. You might see them once a week, once a month, or even less, and not feel lonely in between.

So aim for balance. Learn to enjoy your own company. Think of it as a time when you're free to develop solo interests that you really enjoy. As long as it's your *choice,* and you are not using busyness as a defence against loneliness, there's nothing wrong with doing things on your own.

If you are alone, and it's *not* by choice, do some soul searching. The answer might lie in your own hands. Most of us have our own ways of cutting ourselves off, retreating into our shells. When people say they've too much work or not enough money or that their home is too small/untidy/unattractive to invite people to, they often mean that they're happier putting up with the familiar discomfort of loneliness rather than risking the unfamiliar discomfort of breaking new ground.

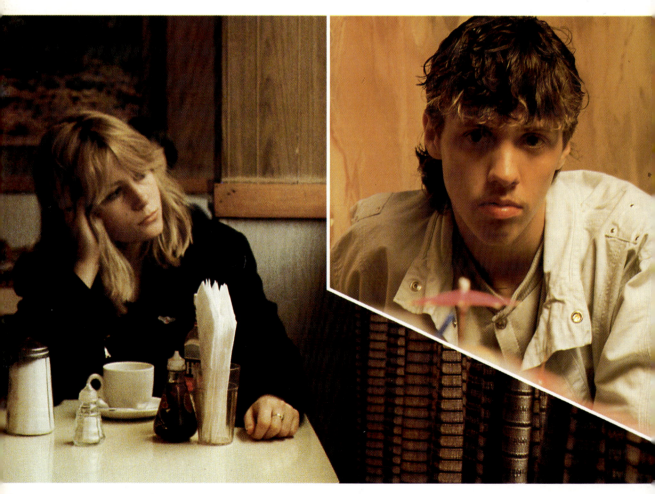

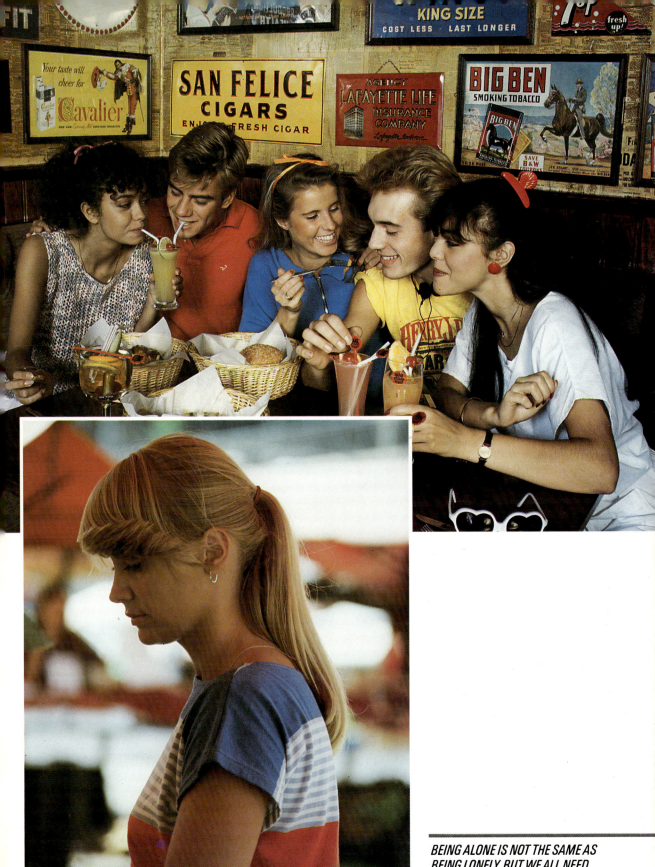

BEING ALONE IS NOT THE SAME AS BEING LONELY, BUT WE ALL NEED PEOPLE SOME TIMES.

If you recognize that loneliness is a problem for you, try to coax yourself out of negative feelings. Don't think 'I won't phone so-and-so because he/she won't want to hear from me'. Don't reject yourself. Phone them. If they don't want to talk to you, or if they don't warm up in the course of the conversation, then *they* are doing the rejecting, not you, and you can cross them off your list. But most people like to feel wanted and remembered. It's flattering.

And don't tell yourself it's not *worth* socializing with people unless they're bosom friends. Being too critical of others is one of the marks of the loner. It's always possible that casual friends, even if they're not socially riveting, will turn into good friends. Take the initiative and arrange for a few of you to meet — in a pub, or in your home if it's convenient. This is the way friendships snowball. If others follow your lead you'll soon have a largish pool of friends, multiplying your chances of developing more intimate relationships.

Shyness

Loneliness is often made worse by shyness. Many of us panic when we're faced with a new social situation, like a job interview or entering a roomful of strange people. Our hands will shake and go clammy, we'll stand rooted to the spot, not knowing what to say...

Yet shyness can be an attractive quality. The modest violet is a more attractive species than the bold sunflower if for no other reason than that people are curious about what is *not* on display. Few of us warm to over-confident, brash individuals who seem to take every social situation in their stride. Most people would agree that there's more satisfaction to be gained from drawing people out than shutting them up.

> '*If they're nice people it doesn't matter in the least if they're shy. The rest of us do too much talking anyway, so it's a relief if there's someone a bit quieter. If someone's obviously shy, you could help them along, but if they're really cold and stand-offish, if they just don't show they're friendly, nobody will bother to be friendly to them.*' HANNAH

What makes us shy? Often shy people have a low opinion of themselves and of how others will judge them. They feel they're not very interesting or witty or attractive. Shyness is their defence mechanism. By not opening their mouths to speak, they avoid making a fool of themselves and by not putting themselves on display, they don't run the risk of looking silly. By hiding themselves away, they don't get noticed, which confirms their belief that they weren't worth noticing in the first place. They save others the bother of rejecting them by rejecting themselves first. We're back to self-rejection again!

Actually shy people, because of their sensitivity, often have a lot to offer. Their shyness is protecting their vulnerability, but it's also denying them the chance to overcome it. The only way to learn from our mistakes is to make some, and learn not to be too ruffled by them. Slowly, little by little, it dawns on us that we *can* take social risks, because when we do the results are not too devastating.

One way to overcome shyness is to ask yourself; 'What effect is my shyness (self-rejection) having on others?' In trying to protect yourself from rejection you are probably sending out rejection messages to them. The signals that go with shyness — lowered eyelids, avoidance of eye contact, muttered attempts at conversation, monosyllabic responses — are also those which tell people you are not interested in them.

It often helps to admit being shy, particularly at parties or large gatherings. You'll find bolder souls quite happy to act as social shields. Or work up your courage by talking to familiar faces first. Just watching other people can also help.

> '*I made two friends early on who were really loud, but really nice and friendly. Through going around with them I lost my shyness. You couldn't be shy with people like that around. I saw how well they got on with everyone. They didn't care what they said and people still liked them.*' NICK

Useful opening gambits

You have to say *something* to break the ice, to break out of your shell of shyness. You don't want to sound daft, but nor do you have to say something worthy of Plato or Bertrand Russell. Remind yourself that you have been on this planet long enough to have plenty of views and feelings to air. And really try to be interested in the person you're talking to — that alone is usually enough to relax you and stop you panicking. And a few slow, deep breaths won't do any harm either. And once the ball is rolling, your interest in the other person and theirs in you should do the rest. So how do you begin those vital opening gambits?

It may be cold comfort now, but most people become less shy as they get older. As our experience of people grows, we have a more solid foundation on which to base our feelings about ourselves. The feedback we get from lots of different people gives us a pretty realistic idea of what our social potential is; until we have received that feedback it may be difficult to feel at ease with the kind of image we're presenting. Later in life you may wish you could revive those fluttery, nervous feelings that once caused such anguish!

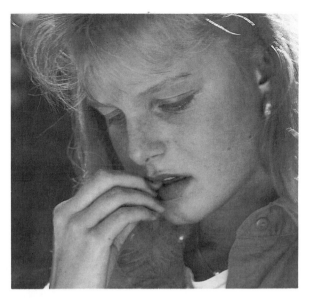

SHY PEOPLE OFTEN HAVE THEIR OWN ATTRACTION: A THOUGHTFULNESS AND SENSITIVITY THAT NEEDS TO BE DRAWN OUT. HOWEVER, IT'S WORTH MAKING THE EFFORT TO OVERCOME EXTREME SHYNESS WHICH CAN BE A REAL SOCIAL DISABILITY.

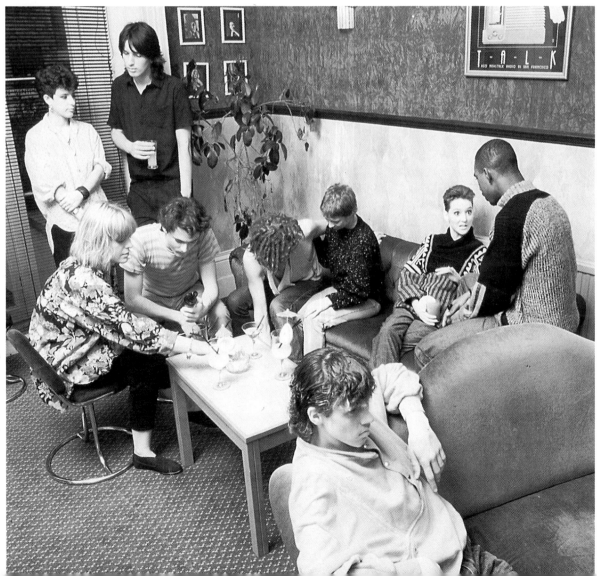

Opening Gambits _____

Let's suppose you're on the brink of some unfamiliar social situation; you're at a party, perhaps, or with a group of people you don't know too well. Your knees are knocking, your palms are clammily clutching your glass, and you'd do anything for the chance to beat a retreat! How do you cope? Some of us have more of a natural flair for dealing with people than others, admittedly, but there are very few individuals who are so confident that they can take every social event in their stride. Getting on with people involves skills which can be learnt by even the shyest amongst us. Inside every introvert there's an extrovert trying to get out.

■ **Try to look and feel positive.** Don't give out looks which apologize for existing. Look as if you know you've something to offer. If it's a party, glance around, choose who you think you might like to talk to and then move in. If you're in a smaller group or you're one to one, don't be afraid to be the one who sets the ball rolling. The others will secretly thank you for it.

■ **Don't plan conversations.** A few prepared one-liners are good to have as stand-bys, but if you think up a dialogue in advance, it's likely to come out sounding stilted. Rehearsing lines reckons without the other person's responses. Saying the first thing that comes into your head isn't always such a disaster. So try to be spontaneous.

■ **Ask open questions.** Avoid those which lead to dead end yes/no answers, 'Do you like…?' 'Have you been to…?', these are dialogue stoppers. Questions like 'What do you think of…?' 'How do you feel about…?', invite ideas and opinions and are less likely to land you up against conversational brick walls.

■ **Put yourself over effectively.** *How* you say something will have just as much effect on your listener as *what* you say, so say it as if it's worth saying. Don't mumble or mutter; by speaking inaudibly or softly, you're almost declaring yourself not worth listening to. Speak loud

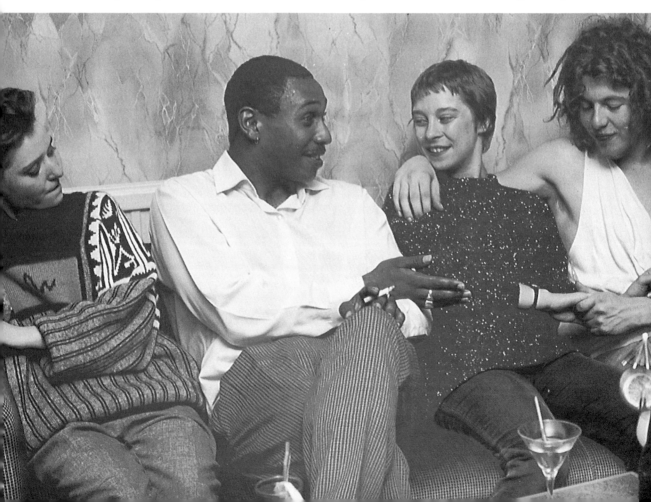

enough for the other person to hear and you probably won't be interrupted.

■ **Learn to link.** Develop a dialogue rather than delivering monologues. Good conversations are more like ping-pong than pinball. If people keep hitting the ball but no one passes it back, you eventually run out of balls. Listen to what people are saying and pick up on it.

■ **Learn to listen.** Every performance needs an audience. There are plenty of people who can talk on effortlessly and those who worry about their lack of conversation often forget how dependent they are on the talkers. Good listeners encourage the talkers by nodding recognition, by making direct eye contact and by leaning towards them. They don't stifle yawns, let their eyes stray or change the subject. They also offer feed-back by constantly picking up on what the other person said, perhaps paraphrasing the last remark, 'You got the job, then?'

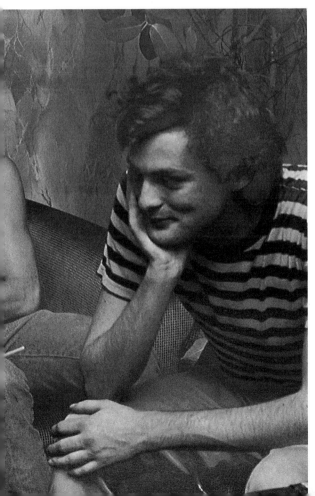

Some dos and don'ts

There are many constructive things you can do to increase your chances of meeting up and making out. Here are some of them.

■ **Don't count on all the desirable specimens of the human race materializing on cue.** Not meeting someone at the disco you've dressed up to the nines for can be a total let-down, but meeting them where you least expect to can be a wonderful bonus.

■ **Do get out and about.** Statistically speaking, you're more likely to meet friends when you're out and about than when stuck at home on your own! People often think that finding a soulmate is a matter of luck — 'Oh, she just happened to be in the right place at the right time' — but for every time you're in the right place there will probably be ninety-nine times when you aren't.

■ **Don't go out with the idea firmly fixed in your head that this time you're going to meet the one and only!** Nine times out of ten you'll be disappointed. Tell yourself that your aim is to sharpen up your social skills and increase your circle of friends.

■ **Do be yourself when you meet people.** The great danger of not being yourself is that you'll never find out if people like you as you are. The chances are that they will.

■ **Don't waste time on someone who really doesn't return your feelings.** There are other pebbles on the beach which may be far more interesting when you turn them over.

■ **Do take a few chances.** Imagine the best possible outcome of your riskier-than-usual behaviour, and also the worst. And weigh the chances of the best happening rather than the worst. If the pay-off looks promising, go ahead.

SOME PEOPLE ARE BORN MIXERS IN, AND THERE'S NO REASON WHY THE REST OF US SHOULDN'T LEARN SOME TIPS FROM THEM.

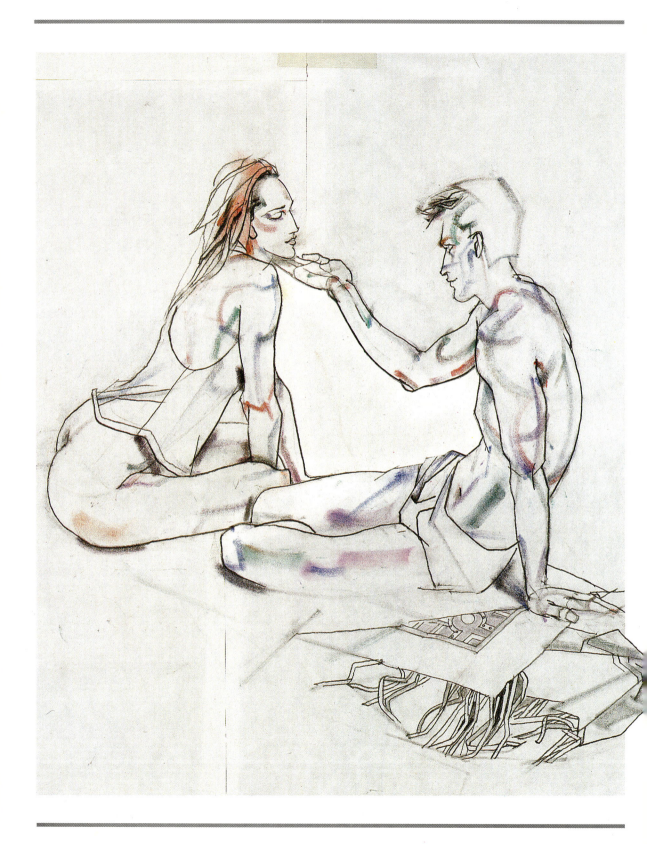

4
But is it love?

How do you recognize the Real Thing? For anyone who's ever experienced it, the signs are unmistakable. Your pulse races, your heart palpitates and you've got a permanent attack of butterflies in the pit of your stomach. You go off your food, you're too excited to sleep, and you sit around waiting for the phone to ring.

'It's a nice feeling. It makes you happier, you feel much better. You see things differently — in a better light. Everything seems easier, you do more things and you do them better. There's also a feeling you can trust someone, someone you can take your problems to and share them with. You can't wait to see each other and you get ridiculously excited and nervous, colly-wobbly!' SUE

'I wanted to be with her all the time and when we weren't together my mind kept going through all the little details of when we last were. I could get down to work OK but even when I was concentrating on other things there was this vague sense at the back of my mind that something about life was different. There wasn't anything I didn't like about her. I think that's honest. Little things I don't like in other people didn't bother me about her.' MARK

'I'd have done anything for him. That sounds terrible doesn't it? Little womanish. But I felt really generous towards him in a way that I hadn't felt towards anyone before. I wanted to know absolutely everything about him, including — no especially! — who he'd been out with, and I got madly jealous if he told me!' CHRISSY

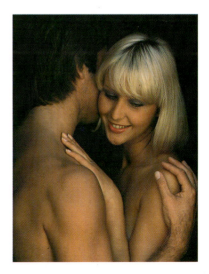

'Excitement really, and an unreal feeling. Ordinary things on my mind stopped worrying me. I was much friendlier and I smiled more. People said I looked different — well and happy. I was completely out of control when I was with her — dangerous, I suppose. I haven't lost those feelings but I think I've become more realistic.' DILLON

These are the dizzy heights of love — the whole stomach-churning, heart-pounding thing, the grand emotion that poets since time began have waxed lyrical about. But there's also a down-to-earth, scientific explanation for these feelings. In fact 'sexual chemistry' is not a bad description of the forces at work between two people madly in love. During the sexual wooing process, certain chemicals (not unlike adrenaline, the 'fight or flight' hormone which flushes through our system at times of emergency) are released which tell the brain to put our reflexes into overdrive. This is why the first symptoms of love feel uncomfortably like the sensations you would get before going hang gliding, making a wedding speech or sitting an exam.

These chemicals act in a similar way to amphetamines or pep pills. Energy levels soar and so do feelings of elation and self-confidence, so that ordinary mortals start to feel like Popeye or Superwoman. Unfortunately, sudden deprivation of these spellbinding substances produces equally strong withdrawal symptoms. Falling out or being jilted leaves lovers with that familiar down-in-the-dumps or flat-as-a-pancake feeling. Where previously you felt ten feet tall, you now feel worthless and unattractive

Is this all love is, then, a state of euphoria, exhilarating, addictive, but short-lived? Is this really love? Or is it lust? Or infatuation? Or being in love with the *idea* of being in love? Will it turn into the real, lasting, now-and-forever kind of relationship that endures long after the cloud nine stuff is over?

Notice that *love* is usually a *noun*, a thing. We talk about 'being in love' and 'falling in love', about being 'smitten by love' or 'sick with love'. It's something we get if we're lucky, like winning a lottery or a raffle. We talk rather less often about 'loving' or 'being loved'. When love is a *verb*, it's something we *do*, a skill or an art we practise, something we actively do to others rather than passively receive from them.

Let's take a closer look at this energy-consuming and energy-giving process. We can think of it in terms of three separate stages. One is the development of mutual attraction. Another is the sharing of interests, attitudes and friends. Another is the growth of expectations and commitments. Though, people don't necessarily work through them in this order.

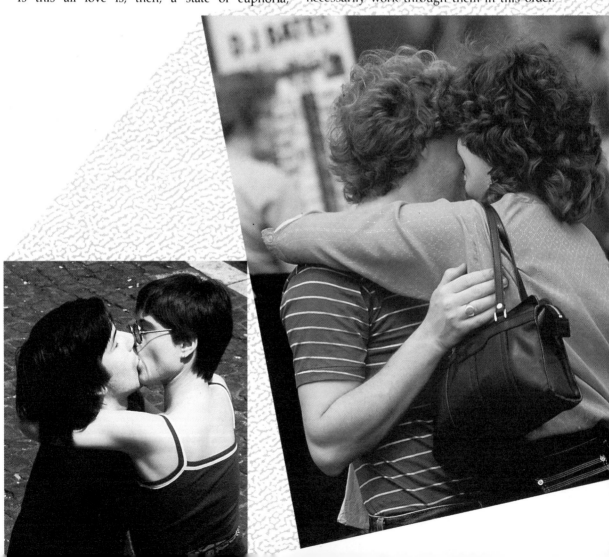

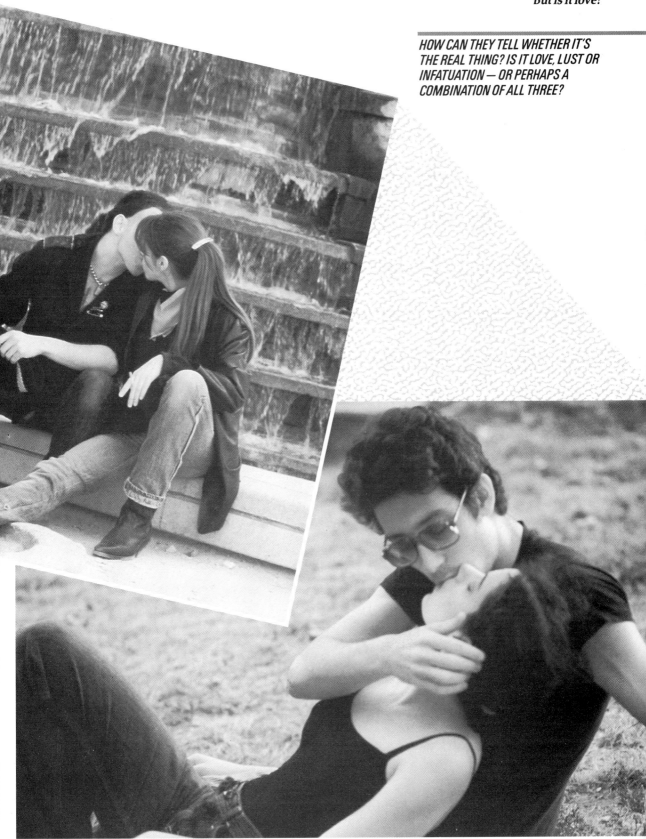

HOW CAN THEY TELL WHETHER IT'S THE REAL THING? IS IT LOVE, LUST OR INFATUATION — OR PERHAPS A COMBINATION OF ALL THREE?

Stage I 'You've got nice earlobes!'_____

There are couples who insist that theirs was love at first sight. They should know. After all, they're the ones who have stuck it out long enough to tell the tale. Those who fell by the wayside cannot apply the same hindsight wisdom. For once a man and woman meet, there has to be some attraction for things to get off the ground. This doesn't mean that either has to have conventionally eye-catching looks, but there has to be *something* there which strikes a sympathetic chord between them.

At this early stage, to paraphrase the White Rabbit in *Alice in Wonderland,* liking what you see is much the same as seeing what you like. Love is not exactly blind, but it does tend to wear highly effective bifocal lenses which filter out the bad points and throw the good ones into sharp focus. At this stage, each partner is an exquisitely flattering mirror to the other. So there's a strong element of vanity involved.

The beginning of a love affair is also marked by quite intense passion, when both parties begin to let down the barriers, share intimate disclosures, and allow themselves to feel close. One of our deepest needs is to overcome feelings of isolation, of being separate from others. Combined with sexual attraction, this new-found intimacy is a very heady potion indeed.

Stage II 'You like pepperoni too?'_____

While you're in the throes of intense physical passion it's difficult, if not impossible, to separate infatuation and lust from something deeper. But gradually, if there's nothing between you but lust or physical craving, you'll get bored and irritated with each other when you're not making love, and eventually an empty and dissatisfied feeling when you are. If there still seems to be some mileage in your love affair once the euphoria stage has run its course, then the stage is set for the next phase of the relationship, and a number of changes are in store.

Firstly, you can expect a change in the emotions you feel. Pleasant though it is, a mutual flattering of vanities isn't enough.

Newly surfacing feelings may seem less intense but they'll be deeper and less self-centred. Loving someone involves caring, respecting and trusting them as well as being turned on by them. You start to feel a real liking for them, and an admiration for what they are and do. You delight in their ups, and feel genuine concern when they're down, and you know they feel the same way about you. Affection and fondness mark the extra emotional dimension at this stage.

At this stage too, your relationship starts to widen out beyond just the two of you. In the early days, feelings are so intense that there's no room for anyone else. But slowly and carefully, you start to pool social networks — you meet each other's workmates, parents and friends. You begin to share interests too. Finding you both like Italian food, discos and Spielberg films can add an exciting new dimension to your friendship.

Sharing friends, interests and attitudes won't shore up a relationship in which two people are basically bored or incompatible with one another, but if you've enough going for you, this broader base helps to cement the bond between you.

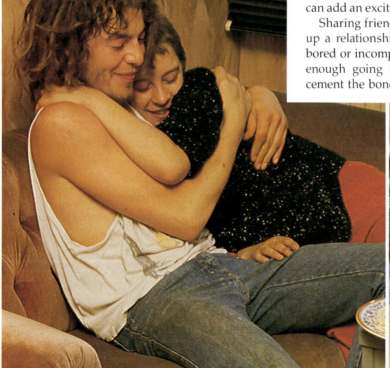

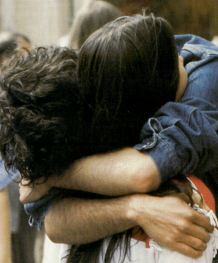

Stage III 'Build me a castle'_____

There's no guarantee that couples who get through the first two hurdles will make it to the finishing post. But as they develop a deeper bond of love, they start to expect (and want to give) some degree of commitment to each other. This commitment marks the next major milestone in the relationship. Up till now you've been a law unto yourselves, love was entered into freely and without obligations. But as you both invest stronger feelings in the relationship, you'll want to feel there's some security.

From now on, you'll find yourself developing some fairly definite expectations about the way you'll both behave. Some of these may not be put into words. There may be an expectation of exclusivity, for example, that you should both be faithful to each other and not date anyone else. There may be an expectation of durability, of lastingness, that the relationship will not be broken off lightly.

Some of these expectations may concern more concrete commitments, like living under the same roof or pooling your finances. This puts the relationship on a totally different footing. Before, there was nothing concrete to support it; it was free to stand or fall, depending only on how well the feelings supported it.

If these faded then so did the relationship. But when you start to build a more durable framework, outside and beyond feelings, the relationship becomes far more difficult (and more painful) to break up. Provided there's no gap or conflict between love and commitment — as there can be if one of you is pressurizing for commitment faster than the other — having some sound external support can help you over a sticky patch, and having got through it, the bond between you may be all the stronger.

THERE'S A LOT OF DIFFERENCE BETWEEN THE 'HEADY' STATE OF A NEW RELATIONSHIP AND THE 'STEADY' STATE OF A MORE MATURE ONE. ONE THING IS VERY OBVIOUS, THOUGH: TWO PEOPLE WHO ARE COMPLETELY OBSESSED WITH ONE ANOTHER ARE OBLIVIOUS TO THE WORLD AROUND THEM.

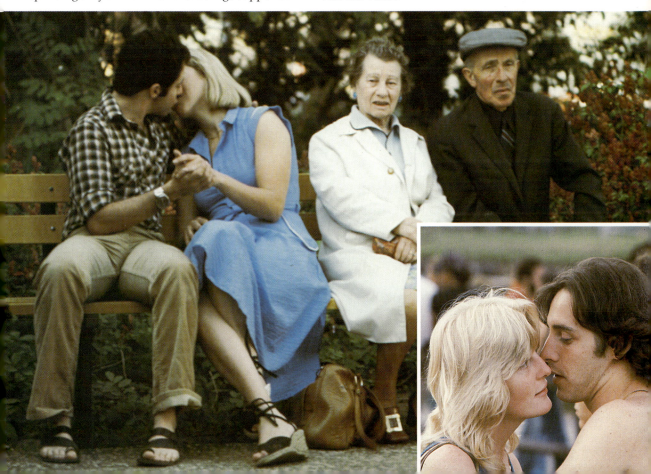

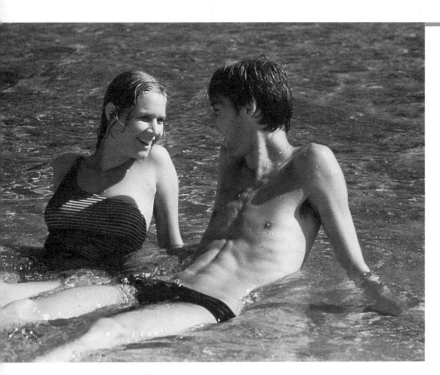

THERE'S PLENTY OF TIME BETWEEN DATING AND MATING TO TRY OUT DIFFERENT RELATIONSHIPS.

Getting stuck at the fences

There is nothing inevitable about moving through these stages. Learning to love is a highly personal thing. People skip stages, reverse the order, or get stuck somewhere along the line. Lust and infatuation *can* mark the start of something permanent and long term, but when we are young they can just as easily be replaced by a new relationship.

A major difference between initial infatuation and a more permanent state of loving is the size of the element of fantasy in the first and the strength of the element of reality in the second. The ability to move from fantasy to reality, to select a mate not according to pipe dreams and wild imaginings but according to what he or she really is, is important in developing a capacity to love, and it comes very much with maturity.

Young girls often have quite passionate feelings which, for want of suitable real life figures, they fix on fantasy objects like pets and pop stars. Boys are somewhat luckier because by the time they go through the same stage, usually a couple of years later, there are some real flesh and blood partners around. But neither sex makes the switch from fantasy to reality overnight. Both tend to have unrealistic expectations of their partners for some time to come.

Nor is it simply a question of age. Some people spend their whole life looking for the ideal mate instead of accepting people for what they are. Since human paragons are few and far between, they are doomed to suffer many disappointments.

If you're finding it difficult to get past the romance/infatuation stage, it's probably because you're not yet able to accept weaknesses, blemishes and imperfections in either yourself or others. You may be so insecure that only the first flush of love will give you a flattering enough picture of yourself to help you overcome your poor self-image. When you're faced with hard, painful or ugly realities, you tend to short-circuit, go back to base and start from scratch with a new partner — that's the only way you can create satisfying images all over again.

The same goes for the move from Stage II to Stage III, from affection and sharing to commitment. You may feel you're too young or haven't had enough experience of life to make the transition, but there are people who, whatever their age, find it difficult to make long-term commitments. Again the cause may be deep-seated feelings of inadequacy or insecurity. By not committing yourself to a partner, you are protecting your fragility.

Sexual love

Love and sex don't automatically go together. Passionate love may not have anything to do with sex. People can love God, their neighbour or the cause of peace; they can love their fellow men and women, without lusting after them. There's much more in the concept of love — feelings of affinity, solidarity, tenderness and fondness — than simply sexual satisfaction.

Similarly, sex may not and often doesn't have anything to do with love. On one level, sexual desire is another physical urge, like hunger and thirst, which our bodies strive to relieve and satisfy. So it's certainly possible to have sex without love, though it's likely to be a rather cool and mechanical affair.

Sexual feelings are said by some to debase love, to drag down our more sensitive and refined feelings. Others hold that it is perfectly possible for two people who have affection for each other to enjoy sex together without permanent involvement, provided they both understand and accept the basis of the relationship, and provided that they treat each other with care and respect.

So sexual attraction and love are not always one and the same, though they shouldn't be thought of as completely separate feelings. They can exist without each other, but they're much richer and stronger when they're together. The problem is that sexual love is often experienced as being a complete fusion or 'one-ness' with another person. While two people are making love they may feel a closeness which is difficult to distinguish from love or from the heady experience of falling in love. If lovemaking doesn't lead on to love, it may leave the two of them feeling further apart than they were before. With their illusions gone, their feelings of being used may turn to anger and hate.

Your capacity to love: the parent factor

Marriage used to be considered too important an institution to exist merely for romantic union. In Europe and America until the turn of the century, (and even today in those societies where marriages still tend to be arranged), couples were matched up by their parents, and on the whole fairly realistically. Paupers didn't marry princes, and duchesses didn't marry doormen. A suitor was judged by his family background, the size of his income, and even his physical fitness — whether he loved his bride-to-be or she loved him was secondary. Love followed marriage if the couple was lucky, but there were no guarantees, and it wasn't considered of any great importance. Of course, people did fall in love despite the conventional wisdom. Fair damsels *did* swoon, and young swains *were* brought to their knees, but all this was thought of as a sickness likely to pave the way for marital disaster rather than a solid foundation for a lifelong partnership.

Today we tend to think that falling in love is a sufficient basis for marriage, or at least for a long-term relationship. The important thing is the intensity of our emotions! This is full-blown, romantic love, as featured in women's magazine stories, pulp fiction and teenage love and romance stories.

Romantic love has a natural time span; it tends to wilt and fade when the going gets tough, when hard, cold practicality intrudes. Sad to say, there is probably no other concept which raises hopes quite as high, leads to quite such tremendous expectations, and which fails quite so regularly — which is why we have probably said enough about it! Many romantic unions burn out a lot quicker than partnerships entered into more prosaically.

Whether we can show love as adults depends very much on two things: how much love our parents gave us and how they showed it, and our opinion of our own worth. Children who receive a lot of physical love — a lot of cuddling and fondling — usually grow up to be more sensuous adults than those whose parents were cold and aloof.

In a sense, the love a parent gives to a child is totally unique. It doesn't need to be deserved, it doesn't need to be returned, and it doesn't always depend on the child being well-behaved, unselfish, kind and thoughtful. Children are often none of these things — they grab, throw tantrums and behave exactly as the mood takes them — but they still get a lot of love.

It's a huge privilege to be loved in this way, and it is unlikely to happen again. For the rest of our lives we have to earn love. Gradually this dawns on us as we grow up. We stop being so self-centred, start thinking about other people, and begin to develop skills of loving as well as being loved.

Some individuals never manage to grasp this. A man stuck in the unconditional phase of love constantly looks for mother figures in his girlfriends and expects them to pander to his every whim; a woman stuck in this phase will, in the same way, be looking for father figures. Both of them will find it difficult to make their adult needs felt. They'll expect them to be intuitively and automatically met, as they were throughout their childhood.

We all grow up carrying the child part of us around inside. It's the charming, fun-loving, pleasure-seeking, creative bit of us inside the adult shell, which is logical, reasonable and sensible. When we want a break from the demands and rigours of being grown-up we let the child in us out to play. Hence the nursery names lovers give each other — 'Piggly', 'Do-do', 'Boodums'. But both partners should take turns to play the child and the adult. A relationship in which one partner is always the parent and the other is always the child hits the rocks when the 'child' eventually 'grows up' — or when the 'parent' wants to revert!

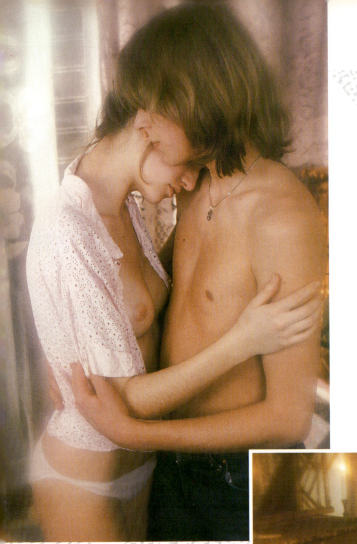

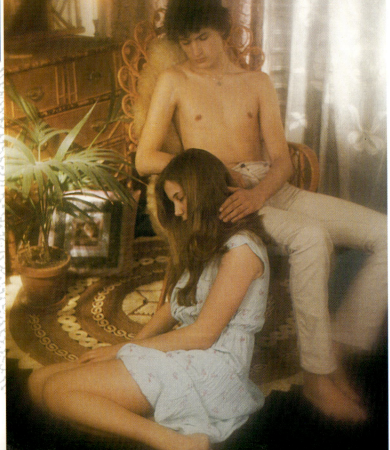

60

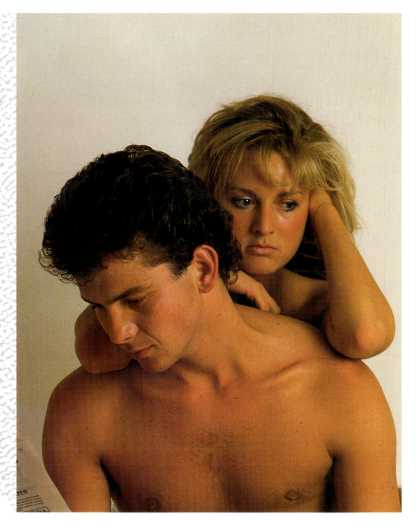

How much do you like yourself?

Self-love is usually seen as an undesirable trait, best avoided. We don't say of someone 'he loves himself' in a kindly spirit. We mean that he is narcissistic and self-centred, too busy loving himself to love others. Truly selfish people are interested only in themselves, want everything for themselves, feel pleasure not in giving but in taking, or only give in order to get. They view the world and the people in it as thoroughly exploitable.

It's easy to fall into the trap of confusing self-love with selfishness. It may sound strange, but selfish people suffer not from too much self-love but from too little. They grab all the goodies for themselves because they feel too unlovable to receive them as a natural right. It is true that selfish people are incapable of loving others, but they're incapable of loving themselves too. So selfishness and self-love, far from being the same thing, are actually opposites.

By contrast, love of self and love for others are inextricably intertwined. We have to love *ourselves* before we can start to love others. This means knowing ourselves, establishing an identity, developing a strong sense of self and believing in ourselves. Some people develop a strong identity comparatively early, in childhood even. Others don't manage to do it until they're in mid-life, and a minority never do. Yet a strong identity is an essential ingredient in learning to love others.

If you don't think highly enough of yourself, you're always going to sell yourself short. You send out messages which say 'Heaven knows why you're in love with *me*'. And perhaps you're doing it so convincingly that your partner ends up wondering the same, and the affair fizzles out. Or your other tactic might be to put your partner down all the time; what you're really doing is cutting him or her down to size to line up with your own self rating. Very destructive.

How high is your self-esteem?

Do you constantly question your worth? Or are you brimful of confidence? How far you agree or disagree with some of the statements below might give you some clues as to how confident you are. Circle the number which best expresses your degree of agreement. For example, in the third statement, if you're often accused by others of needing a soap box, you'd circle 9, if you sometimes have a lot to say and at other times nothing, you'd circle 5, and if you feel you're very mouse-like, then you'd circle 1. Add up the score of the circled numbers.

STATEMENT		STATEMENT
I have terrible problems making decisions. I seem to blow with the wind and change my mind by the minute	1 2 3 4 5 6 7 8 9	If I make my mind up about something, I don't often change it
If people criticize me it can make me upset and depressed	1 2 3 4 5 6 7 8 9	Things other people say about me don't bother me much. If they're not complimentary I just simply ask myself why they feel the need to pull me to pieces — are they jealous, for example
I tend to keep my ideas and opinions quiet in case they get challenged. I find it difficult to defend them	1 2 3 4 5 6 7 8 9	I'm a great one for sounding off about something. I may not be always right but I do feel my ideas are worth stating
I have terrible difficulty *finishing* things. My ideas seem OK at the start but my resolve seems to peter out somewhere along the line	1 2 3 4 5 6 7 8 9	If I start something I always see it through to the end
Unless I really know people well, I behave in a very reserved way towards them. I'd be nervous of showing too many feelings at the start	1 2 3 4 5 6 7 8 9	When I first meet people I go overboard to really project myself. I suppose some people could complain that I'm a little overbearing and forward
I always pay more attention to my partner than myself when I'm making love	1 2 3 4 5 6 7 8 9	When I'm making love I concentrate more on my pleasure than on that of my partner
I have to admit I do bitch or gossip about someone. Picking out other people's imperfections makes me feel better myself	1 2 3 4 5 6 7 8 9	I rarely talk in a bad way about other people. We've all got weaknesses as well as strengths but I find people's good points more interesting

STATEMENT		STATEMENT
I often have nagging doubts about whether my partner might find someone else more attractive and interesting than me	1 2 3 4 5 6 7 8 9	Jealousy is not really something that bothers me. I usually feel quite secure in my relationships
I tend to blow with the wind a bit in discussions. It's more important to me that people like me than it is for me to make some particular point	1 2 3 4 5 6 7 8 9	I don't easily change my opinions. If other people think differently this doesn't alter the way I think
I don't feel I'm confident enough to be stretched too far. I tend to stick to fairly easy and undemanding people and jobs	1 2 3 4 5 6 7 8 9	I enjoy challenges in my jobs and in my relationships

How did you score? _____

Fewer than 25 points You have a very fragile ego which must be extremely difficult to live with. You probably go in fear of it being knocked and bruised and this may prevent you doing a lot of things you'd like to do. Your self doubts and insecurity probably also prevent other people from really getting to know you and make you especially vulnerable to odd thoughtless remarks. To develop a more solid sense of your own worth, you need to find a supportive environment in which people who appreciate you can give you really positive feelings about yourself, which you'll *eventually* believe in.

25-50 points

You too are beset by feelings of insecurity, but you have a more solid sense of self which prevents your feelings about yourself vacillating quite so wildly. To be really comfortable, though, you still need to develop a slightly thicker skin, together with the capacity to fail, or suffer defeats sometimes, without being really thrown by them. An *element* of self doubt though is worth clinging on to, since it does make us keep on trying.

50-75 points

You are not very easily shaken, can cope with most situations and rise to most challenges. You are probably used as a prop by others because your inner strength is tempered by just enough vulnerability to make you sensitive and sympathetic.

More than 75 points

You are obviously rocklike in your feelings of self confidence, but are you sure your sense of security isn't perhaps bordering on stubbornness and a refusal to bend to other people. If people are completely indifferent to other people's opinions there's a risk that they bulldoze their way through life, trampling on toes and denting self-images. A little more attention to other people's needs would make you a more sensitive person to live with.

The end of an affair

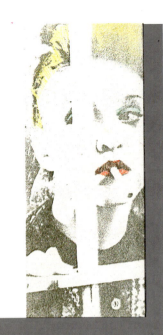

The outlook that only one single person in the world is right for us is not very helpful. There are any number of people you can live happily ever after with provided you've got what it takes to live happily. So though it seems like the end of the world at the time, breaking off a love affair is something that happens to a lot of us at least once, and perhaps several times.

Especially if it is based on physical attraction rather than common interests and attitudes, a romance can fade quite abruptly. Feelings can up and off with very little warning. But there may be some advance signs that the relationship is wearing thin. Here are some of them.

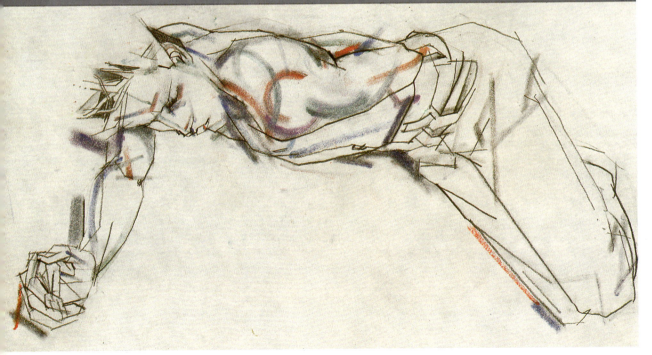

WHEN YOU'RE GETTING OVER A LOVE AFFAIR, DON'T KEEP THE GRIEF TO YOURSELF.

■ **You start being excessively critical of each other,** not in a constructive way, but in a nagging, nit-picking way — she's always losing her keys/never has any cash; he makes unfunny jokes/is always late. Little things bother you which didn't before, and they start to outnumber the things that please you.

■ **You start to feel constricted,** as though you have to report your movements, account for your actions. Your partner seems to be making demands on you that you're not prepared to meet, and you resent it.

■ **Tension levels run high,** it becomes a strain to be together, and the times you spend bickering or at loggerheads start to get longer than the times when you're in harmony.

■ **You get less attentive towards each other.** You phone each other less often and you meet less regularly.

If, for you, the situation seems to have reached the point of no return, there are some things you can do to lessen the blow of telling your partner. Be as positive as possible. Point out how much the relationship has meant to you and how much you've learned from it (assuming you have, of course). There's no point in making promises you can't keep, but if you think you can realistically stay friends, say so.

Of course, it may be you who is receiving the brush-off. If you've already read the signs, the news won't be quite such a bombshell. But when we're in love we often wear blinkers and only after the bad news is broken do we run the tape back and see the incidents that foretold the break.

Getting over it

Accept that you might need weeks or even months, rather than days, to get over the end of a love affair. You need time to grieve, as you would over the death of someone you love. Unrequited love is a miserable state of affairs, so have an indulgent wallow if you feel the need to — much better than keeping your feelings all bottled up. Don't keep it all to yourself either. Choose carefully who to confide in, but then, no holds barred, let it all out. Resist the temptation to spy on your 'ex's' movements by getting friends to play private detective — you're only torturing yourself. Even if you feel you never want to set eyes on a prospective partner again, console yourself with the thought that as one door closes, another opens. Remember that there's one thing to be said for hitting rock bottom — the only possible direction is up!

Sexual etiquette _____

■ **Always reject gently.** For some reason many people refuse a cup of tea with more grace than they would the offer of a date. Remember that it takes quite a lot of courage to ask someone out, so if you give someone the brush off make sure you do so in such a way that it's clear that though *you're* not interested, you're sure that plenty of others would be, and that you're flattered to be asked.

■ **Never stand someone up.** If you've arranged a date, just not turning up is a real coward's way out and is very, very hurtful to the other person's feelings. If you have regrets about the arrangement, phone to make your excuses. Better still, be firm in your refusal in the first place.

■ **Plan to go Dutch.** On a financial note, it's best to assume that you're going Dutch, unless one of you is far better off than the other. This doesn't mean that you can't accept treats now and again, but never think in terms of buying company or having yours bought.

■ **Don't be pushy.** If you're asked out, never assume it's a sexual advance. Don't push the pace either. Never be afraid to say that you don't want your evening out to end in bed.

■ **Don't force decisions.** If there's a decision to be made, always make sure your partner has a *real* choice. Asking someone to stay the night, for example, is not a fair question if you've engineered things in such a way that he or she has missed the last bus.

■ **Let him/her down gently.** If you decide you don't want to see someone again, always phone or meet and say so. Never, never just leave thoughts and feelings in the air. Feeling that you weren't even worth the effort of an explanatory phone call can be *very* damaging to self esteem.

■ **Comparisons are odious.** Never compare someone who is currently special in your life with a previous partner or lover. If the comparison is unfavourable it's obviously insulting, but even if it's favourable, people don't like to be measured against some sort of human yardstick.

■ **Don't take possession of someone too soon.** Be wary of getting closer than you think they can cope with and give them space and time to develop their feelings for you. Watering the plants, making plans to redecorate or answering the phone in someone else's home can feel very intrusive.

■ **Don't act like a vulture.** Swooping in on someone else's partner is an easy way to lose friends. If two people have recently split up, you should be especially wary of appearing to have been watching like a hawk, ready to move in.

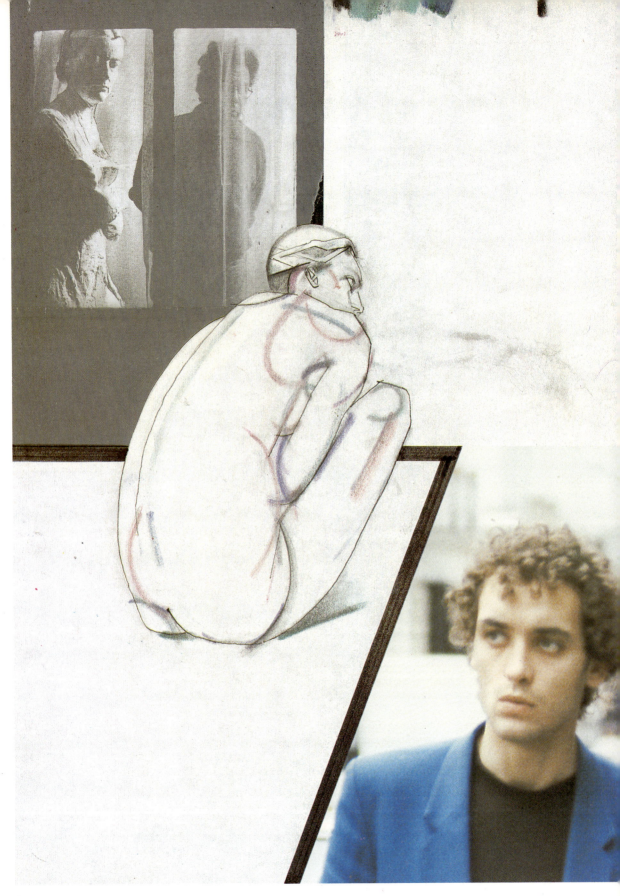

5
Playing safe

Look at any book on love and sex and the chances are you'll find the chapter on birth control much further down the contents list than it is in this one. The reason is obvious — making love is about excitement and pleasure, and birth control is about boring practical realities. All too often, this is the sequence in real life. Sex comes first and contraception is an afterthought. But like it or not, it is a biological fact that if you want to avoid pregnancy, contraceptive planning *must* come *before* sexual experience. So avoid the temptation to skip this chapter.

Contraception and the law

In England, Scotland, Wales and Northern Ireland a person is regarded as medically adult at the age of 16. He or she has the right to professional privacy and the right to decide whether, or what, information should be passed to parents. However, although it is better to involve parents where possible, in cases when this is most difficult doctors are empowered to prescribe contraception to young people under 16, in exceptional circumstances, without parental consent.

It is a responsible act to seek contraceptive advice. If you are met with criticism or lecturing from the doctor you seek advice from, find another doctor. And remember, your parents have almost certainly been using some form of birth control for years, or you would be one of at least ten children! They are far more likely to applaud your responsibility than disown you for wanting, or having, a sex life.

Some typical attitudes to contraception

Doctors are all too aware that most people making their first appointment for birth control are already having sex and have probably been panicked into coming by a 'near miss'. Of course they would rather see the near misses than those who don't get a second chance. But they're all too familiar with a variety of plaintive cries.

'We'd had sex a lot and she didn't get pregnant.'

But she did in the end. If you take a chance you *may* be lucky, but that will almost certainly encourage you to take more chances. Eventually your luck runs out and it's likely to be sooner rather than later. Mother Nature has the odds stacked heavily in her favour when it comes to keeping the human race going. The chances of getting pregnant increase alarmingly at certain times in the woman's monthly cycle: if you make love just before ovulation

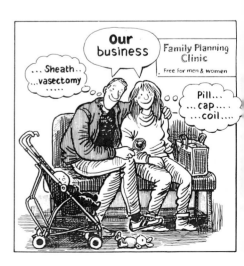

67

they increase to 1 in 3, and on the day of ovulation to 1 in 2 — a real 'heads or tails' gamble. If a hundred fertile, healthy couples with normal sexual appetites have unprotected sex over a period of a year, ninety of them are likely to be prospective parents at the end of it.

'I didn't know how to go about it.'

Most of us today have some knowledge of birth control methods, but asking for them can still be a problem. Asking for contraceptives means admitting to someone else that you're sexually experienced, or at least planning to be. More important, it means admitting this to yourself, and sex is still steeped in enough guilt to make this difficult for many of us. It's not easy to tell the doctor who treated your measles that you now have a sex life. It may also take some courage to face an assistant across a counter and ask for sheaths. It may cost you some embarrassment and loss of face, but what are they against the much higher costs of an unwanted pregnancy?

'For me, sex was something that just happened. I couldn't have sat down beforehand and thought it all out.'

Seeing sex as something completely spontaneous

means that at least we can't be accused of stage-managing the whole thing. Besides, most of us prefer to think of love-making as having more to do with passion and uncontrollable feelings than with cucumber-cool forward planning. In romantic films and novels heroines never untwine themselves to fit caps nor do heroes fumble about with sheaths! Yet there's nothing very romantic about unplanned pregnancy. If two people can discuss together what they're going to do to prevent pregnancy, it probably won't be a very passionate discussion, but it does show that they care.

'All the methods I'd heard about seemed risky. I thought, why bother?'

Admittedly, no one has come up with the perfect contraceptive, but wishful thinking never stopped anyone getting pregnant. No method is guaranteed 100 per cent reliable, but *not* using a method is 100 per cent *unreliable*. To cut the risks to a minimum, it's worth putting some time and effort into considering not only which method will suit you best, but which one you'll *use* best. However safe a method is in theory, in practice it's only as good as its user. Use the chart on page 71 to help you.

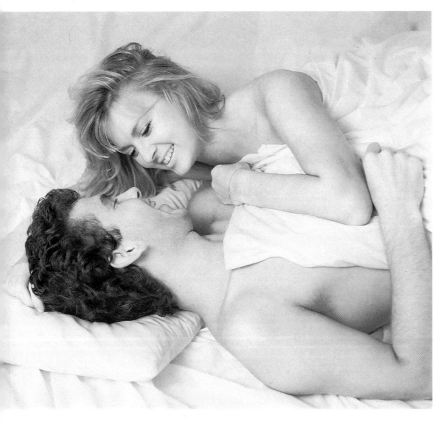

MAKING LOVE IS A JOYOUS ACTIVITY BUT YOU SHOULD ALWAYS REMEMBER TO TAKE PRECAUTIONS. CONTRACEPTION FIRST: LOVEMAKING SECOND.

A method for you

There's nothing very tempting about taking pills every day or using sheaths. On the other hand, it's worth bearing in mind that the vast majority of unplanned pregnancies occur not because contraceptive methods are unromantic, or because they fail or are carelessly used, but because people are so often caught off guard — they get themselves into sexual relationships before they've had a chance to prepare.

If you're in a steady relationship, then the realization that sometime or other you're going to make love will be gradual enough to give you time to plan ahead, time to find the method you are going to use best. Most books on birth control and sex give plenty of information about the risks of pregnancy, the safety of each method and its side-effects, and this one is no exception — you'll find most of this information in this chapter. Though all these facts are vitally important, there is also some information which only *you* can put into your decision-making. The details of your lifestyle will be essential in helping you make your choice, so it's worth asking yourself a few questions before you take the plunge.

'Who is going to take precautions?'

This will depend very much on the relationship between you and your partner, and on the discussions between you about what would be best. But whether the method is used by the woman or the man, THE RESPONSIBILITY SHOULD BE A JOINT ONE. Responsibility for remembering should lie with both of you and any health risks or inconveniences should be understood and accepted by both of you. One of you should not enjoy risk-free sex at the expense of the other's peace of mind.

'How often am I likely to make love?'

This is a vital factor in deciding which method to use. If your lovemaking is more of a monthly treat than a nightly marathon, then you should consider whether it's really worth using a 'systemic' method, one which affects your whole body all of the time (the pill is systemic). You don't leave the central heating on all day if you're only in for lunch! If you don't get the chance to be together very often, or if your sexual appetite is not particularly large, you'll probably find a one-off method — like the sheath or the cap — a better bet.

'Where will I make love?'

In other words, how much privacy and what sort of facilities will you have? Ideally, lovemaking should not be a hasty hole-in-the-corner business, but a relaxed and leisurely event in comfortable surroundings. Having to share living quarters can make this difficult. So if you don't have undisturbed access to a bathroom to fit a cap or diaphragm and you don't feel comfortable about making it part of your lovemaking, then an alternative method may suit you better.

'What will suit my lifestyle?'

Some methods — the mini-pill for example — depend on your being able to attend to them at very nearly the same time every day. This is fine if you have a well-regulated lifestyle which finds you in roughly the same place at the same time each day. If not, the risk of forgetting is fairly high.

'Will I like the method?'

You won't know until you try, of course, but you might have some initial preferences. It's important to be honest with yourself about these; the more comfortable you feel with a method, the better you'll use it. Experts distinguish between 'user failure' and 'method failure' and generally agree that the risks of pregnancy have just as much to do with the first as with the second. A method might be safe as houses scientifically, but used wrongly it will be near useless. Your unconscious may be the gremlin here; if you find a method distasteful you may 'forget' to use it. If a woman feels squeamish about exploring the inner recesses of her body, she is unlikely to be a perfect cap or diaphragm user. An aversion to drugs and medication generally will make pill-taking patterns unreliable. Similarly, if a man genuinely finds the sheath distasteful, he will find some excuse for not using it.

'How do I feel about doctors?'

Pills, caps, diaphragms and IUDs (intra-uterine device) have to be prescribed and/or fitted by a doctor. If you don't like the idea of discussing your sex life with or being examined by a doctor, for whatever reason, these methods will not be for you. Better to use a method, like the sheath, which can be purchased and used without consulting a doctor.

Methods of Birth Control

The effectiveness of any method of birth control is most simply expressed in terms of the number of women out of a hundred who would get pregnant using it for a whole year. So a totally safe method — like total chastity, or sterilization — would have a failure rate of 0 out of 100, and a totally unsafe method — like trusting to luck and nothing else — would have a failure rate of 90 out of 100.

The table opposite shows the relative effectiveness of all the methods discussed in this chapter. They fall into various categories: there are hormonal methods, like the pill; barrier methods like the sheath, cap and diaphragm; natural methods, which use the body's natural rhythms; and other methods like the IUD and spermicides.

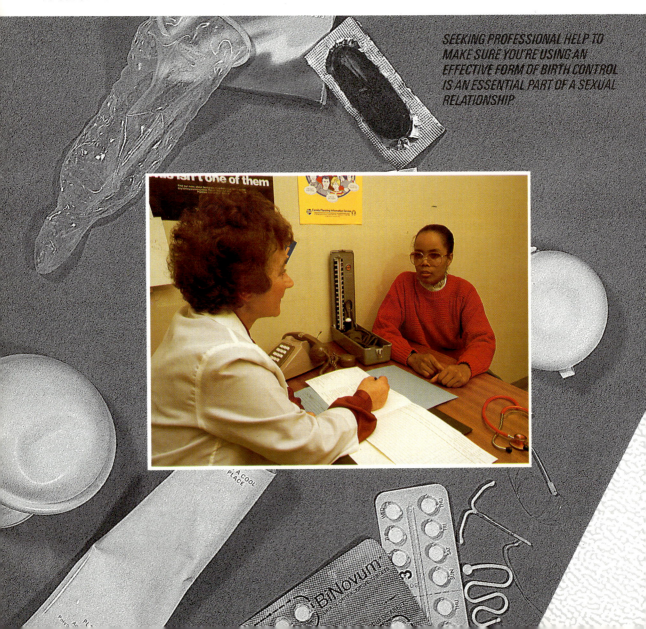

SEEKING PROFESSIONAL HELP TO MAKE SURE YOU'RE USING AN EFFECTIVE FORM OF BIRTH CONTROL IS AN ESSENTIAL PART OF A SEXUAL RELATIONSHIP.

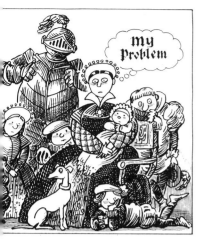
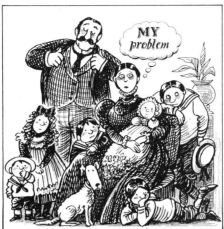
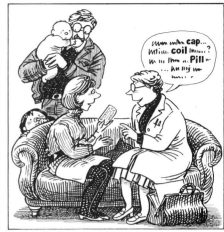

Playing safe: a league table

METHOD	FAILURE RATE (Pregnancies per 100 women using method regularly for 1 year)	EFFECTIVENESS
Combined pill	0.3/100	**over 99%** when correctly used
Mini pill	2/100	**98%** when correctly used
Sheath	3/100	**85-98%** effective
Cap/diaphragm	3/100	**85-97%** effective
IUD	2-4/100	**96-99%** effective
Billings/mucus method	7-15/100	**85-93%** effective
Sponge	15-20/100	**75-91%** effective
Withdrawal Spermicides only	17-25/100	**75-83%** effective
Nothing	90/100	—

Survey

A willingness on the part of young men to share in contraceptive responsibility was revealed by a study carried out by the Health Education Council into men's attitudes towards contraception. A total of 78 per cent of the young men interviewed said they saw contraception as a joint affair; 82 per cent said a man should always ask a girl about contraception before assuming it was all right to have sex; and 79 per cent said that if their girlfriend wasn't protected, then they should wear a sheath. Only 11 per cent said they thought they should leave it to their partners to bring up the business of contraception. Sadly these lofty intentions are not always translated into practice. One third reported that the first time they had sex they didn't take precautions.

The pill

The pill has a huge following among younger women today. It works by making the environment of the womb hostile to sperm and, in the case of the combined pill, by preventing ovulation (egg release) as well. The pill is a 'hormonal' method, as opposed to a 'barrier' or 'natural' method of contraception. It prevents conception in the same way that the body does during pregnancy, by means of hormones.

The combined pill

The combined pill contains two synthetic hormones, oestrogen and progestogen, which are as near one can get in a test tube to the two natural hormones (oestrogen and progesterone) produced by women's bodies to help control the cycle of reproduction. The combination works in two ways. Normally, when the level of natural oestrogen drops, as it does during a period, a signal is sent to the brain which triggers off a process which leads to the release of an egg for fertilization. By artificially boosting the level of this hormone, the combined pill stops this process. No egg, no pregnancy.

Just in case the odd intrepid egg manages to escape the effects of the oestrogen, the other artificial hormone, progestogen, sets to work to make sure it doesn't get fertilized. Progestogen causes the lining of the womb to build up and shed — as it does during menstruation — and also makes the natural secretions at the entrance to the womb much thicker, making it more difficult for sperm to reach the womb. So the combined pill is very much a 'belt and braces' method; it would be difficult, if not impossible, for egg and sperm to survive this assault course and get together.

Researchers are constantly coming up with improved versions of the combined pill. The newest version on the market is the *phasic pill*, which takes into account the ebb and flow of the natural levels of hormones in a woman's body throughout her menstrual cycle, and releases only as much of each hormone as is needed at any one time of the month to prevent pregnancy. For this reason it is essential that the pills are taken in correct order — the packs are coloured to make this easier. The tri-phasic pill has three different strengths of hormone in a monthly pack and the bi-phasic pill has two.

Using the combined pill

The combined pill comes in packets of 21, 22 or 28 pills, with clear instructions on how they should be used. In the case of 21- and 22-day packs, one pill is taken consecutively on each of the 21 or 22 days followed by a break of 7 and 6 days respectively. During the pill-free days you have a 'withdrawal bleed' which may be lighter or shorter than a normal period, but you are still protected against pregnancy during this time. At the end of the pill-free break, you take the first pill of the next month's pack. With the 28-day pack, you take one pill every day without a break, but you can expect to bleed during the last 7 days of the cycle (when you're actually taking 'dummy' or 'reminder' pills).

When you first start taking a course of pills, you may be told to start your first pack in one of two ways. Some doctors recommend taking the first pill on the fifth day of your period, and to use another form of birth control (the sheath, for example) if you make love during the first 14 days of pill-taking. Other doctors advise starting the first pill on the first day of your period, in which case you're protected without any additional precautions from the start of the course.

If you're prescribed one of the newer bi-phasic or tri-phasic pills, you take the first pill on the first day of your period, but you must be sure to take the pills in the right order. They are colour-coded to make this easier.

If you take the pill, you need to get into the habit of taking it at roughly the same time each day. If your pills are next to your toothbrush, they're much easier to remember. If you do miss a pill, take it as soon as you realise, but if you are more than 12 hours late in taking it, you can't be sure that you're protected, so you should take extra precautions for the next 14 days.

The 'mini-pill' or progestogen-only pill

Unlike the combined pill, which contains two female hormones, the mini-pill contains only one, progestogen, and in a smaller dose than the combined pill. This small dose is not usually enough to stop ovulation; the mini-pill relies, for its contraceptive effect, on preventing an egg from being fertilized. It does this by making the mucus at the entrance to the womb thicker and more difficult for sperm to penetrate. The mini-pill may be a good choice for women who experience side-effects with the combined pill, but it can produce slight bleeding between periods (called 'breakthrough bleeding') which can be irritating. It is a less powerful method than the combined pill but taken correctly it is only slighty less reliable.

Using the mini-pill

The higher failure rate of the mini-pill is partly due to users forgetting to take it regularly. To be effective the mini-pill must be taken at the same time (or within an hour either way) every day, and you only have three hours grace if you forget (compared with 12 hours if you forget to take the combined pill). So think carefully: will you be able to stick to this clockwork regime? If you have any doubts, make them known to the person prescribing for you.

You start taking the mini-pill on the first day of your period and you should take additional precautions for the first 14 days of the first pack. You take each course for 28 days, then begin the next one. *Do not worry* if you don't have a period at all; this simply means you are not ovulating. Breakthrough bleeding and spotting may be a problem, but it is not harmful or abnormal. If it upsets you, mention it to your doctor at your next appointment.

Warning!

Some medicines (certain antibiotics, for example) can interfere with the action of the pill, so check with your doctor to find out if the one you're taking has this effect. If it does, go on taking the pill as usual, but use another method of birth control until the end of your course of treatment, and for 14 days afterwards. A bout of sickness or diarrhoea can also prevent absorption of the pill. The rule is, if you've kept your pill down for longer than 3 hours in the case of sickness or 12 hours in the case of diarrhoea, you can consider yourself safe — otherwise, take additional precautions (the sheath, for example) for the next 14 days.

Is the pill safe?

It is now nearly a quarter of a century since the pill first became available and in that time medical researchers have constantly been monitoring its effects. The substances that make the pill effective are powerful drugs and it would be surprising if they didn't have effects other than purely contraceptive ones. Some of these effects may be welcome, others less so. Some are hardly noticeable, others more so. But it's important that pill users should be aware of them.

Something like four out of ten women taking the pill report side-effects which are uncomfortable or irritating. These include feelings of nausea or sickness, headaches, weight gain and, in some cases, mood changes such as depression or a loss of sexual appetite. Mostly these problems clear up after a few months of regular use, but for a few women they may persist long enough to prompt them to abandon the pill in favour of another method. On the credit side, many women find the pill relieves the symptoms of menstruation — their periods become more regular, lighter, less painful, and they experience less premenstrual tension. Making up your mind about the pros and cons of pill use will depend on which of these (if any) affect *you* most.

The pill has also been linked with some more serious side-effects — an increased risk of high blood-pressure and blood clotting in some women, for example. More recently, there have been studies which suggest that more women who take the pill develop cancer of the cervix than those who don't, and that women who start taking the pill very young and continue to do so for a long time may be more likely to suffer from breast cancer. Other studies have shown that the pill may protect users against other diseases, such as cancer of the womb and ovaries, and arthritis.

These studies have to be taken seriously, but we also have to remember that many of the women studied were taking higher-dose pills than are prescribed today. Unfortunately, we'll have to wait another ten or fifteen years before we know what effects today's lower-dose pills are having. But whatever the long-term effects of the pill, we know that the risks are greater if you smoke, if you have high blood-pressure, or if anyone in your family has suffered from heart disease, thrombosis or stroke. Talk these things through with your partner and doctor before you decide whether the pill is the method for you.

If you decide it is, watch carefully for any unusual symptoms — any headaches or fainting, chest or stomach pains, or swellings in leg muscles — and report them to your doctor immediately. Get into the habit, too, of examining your breasts regularly (see page 185) and making sure you have a regular cervical smear (see page 185).

We all have our own personal level of risk tolerance. For some women, any side-effects the pill may have are outweighed by its reliability. If no amount of reassurance gets rid of nagging doubts — and anxiety can be just as harmful as physical side-effects — you should seriously consider an alternative method.

ORAL CONTRACEPTIVES: PACKETS OF PILLS ARE CLEARLY MARKED WITH THE DAYS OF THE WEEK AND THE ORDER IN WHICH THE PILLS SHOULD BE TAKEN.

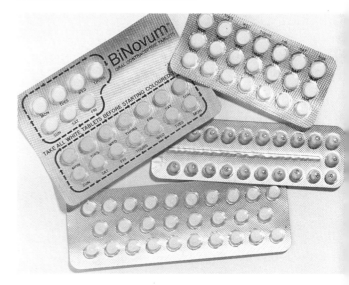

Barrier methods

These are methods that physically prevent the man's sperm from reaching the woman's cervix or womb. The theory is that sperm never get the chance to reach an egg or fertilize it. In practice, this means using the method *every* time you make love.

The sheath

Sheaths suffer from image problems. Not so long ago they were used to prevent sexually transmitted diseases rather than pregnancy, and to some extent the stigma still sticks. They also tend to be linked with furtive adolescent sex; a packet of sheaths tucked into a top pocket has been many a young man's first proud statement that he is sexually experienced (whether he is or not!).

Yet the humble sheath has a lot to recommend it. Currently it is the only method of birth control which can be used by men without the fear of putting paid permanently to their chances of becoming fathers. It is easy to use and has absolutely no side-effects. In fact, sheaths may help to protect both men and women against certain sexually transmitted diseases and may also reduce the risk of cancer of the cervix in women. They are reliable and above all they're easily available. Supplies are free from family planning clinics (though not from your family doctor) and can be obtained quite cheaply and without prescription from chemists and other stores, from hairdressers, and from vending machines in men's lavatories.

Sheaths have gained something of a reputation as 'passion killers' because their use can interrupt lovemaking. Yet, with a bit of imagination, putting them on can become part of foreplay. Manufacturers have certainly put a lot of effort into making them more appealing: modern sheaths come in a variety of shapes, sizes and colours, and some even have raised bumps and ridges to produce more exciting sensations, though it's doubtful whether most people notice the difference!

Using a sheath

A sheath is simply a long tube of latex rubber, sealed at one end, which fits over the erect penis and catches the semen when it is ejaculated, so that sperm don't enter the woman's vagina and can't reach the egg to fertilize it.

The sheath should be rolled carefully onto the penis *after* it has become erect but *before* it makes any contact with the vagina. This is important because some semen can leak from the tip of the penis at an early stage in lovemaking. The last half inch (1cm) of the closed end should be pinched between finger and thumb of the free hand; this leaves room for the semen and makes sure no air is trapped which might cause the sheath to burst. Putting the sheath on can be a joint effort if both parties feel comfortable with the idea, but watch out for fingernails and rings which could snag the fine latex.

After the man has ejaculated but *before* he loses his erection, he holds the rim of the sheath firmly around his penis so that when he withdraws the sheath doesn't slip off, accidentally allowing sperm into the vagina. A sheath should *never* be used more than once. Some couples like to be extra sure and use a spermicide as well as a sheath, but this is not essential, and besides, many sheaths now have a built-in spermicidal agent.

Health risks and the sheath

There are occasional cases of people finding they're allergic to sheaths, either to the rubber or the spermicide, but these are rare and some chemists stock special non-allergenic sheaths.

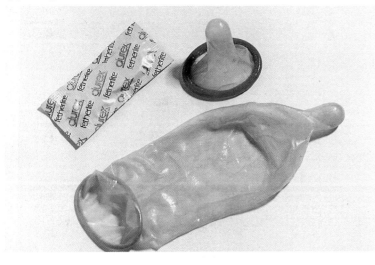

SHEATHS OR CONDOMS: THE ONLY 'REVERSIBLE' METHOD OF CONTRACEPTION WHICH CAN BE USED BY MEN.

The cap and the diaphragm

Women tend to have mixed feelings about using the cap. Disillusioned users will regale you with stories of their caps springing out of their hands and flying across the bathroom. They complain about the mess and the loss of spontaneity in sex. But others swear by the method, and gladly put up with a little inconvenience in return for knowing that they are in no way interfering with the workings of their bodies. The two basic requirements of using a cap or diaphragm properly are firstly, knowing where the cervix is, so that the cap or diaphragm can be fitted over it, and secondly, not feeling squeamish about delving around for it. If you don't feel comfortable about putting your fingers inside yourself, you're probably not going to be a good cap or diaphragm user.

We talk loosely of 'using the cap' when in fact we're talking about two similar but separate methods — *caps* and *diaphragms*. A diaphragm is a shallow dome of rubber mounted on a springy metal rim; correctly inserted into the vagina, it sits upside down over the cervix, the entrance to the womb. A cap is smaller and fits more precisely over the cervix itself.

Both devices work on exactly the same principle as the sheath; they stop sperm reaching the egg and fertilizing it. They do this in two ways. Firstly, the cap or diaphragm forms a barrier between sperm and womb and, secondly, it acts as a container for spermicide which kills off any sperm which manage to find their way around the rim. So it must always be used with spermicide and must always fit as snugly as possible.

How to use a cap or diaphragm

Although you can buy a cap or diaphragm in a chemist's shop without prescription, you must know what size you need and for this a visit to your own doctor or to a doctor at a family planning clinic is essential. At the first appointment a vaginal examination is carried out; then you'll be taught how to insert the cap or diaphragm properly, and probably given one to practise with (though you won't be encouraged to use this during intercourse until you've really mastered it). The two golden rules of using the cap or diaphragm are:

■ Make sure your cap fits. Get it checked every six months, or sooner if you've lost or gained more than 7 lb (3kg) in weight.

■ Remember to use the spermicide properly. Spermicides come in the form of foams, creams, gels or pessaries, but tubes of cream are handiest to use with a cap.

Begin by checking that you can feel exactly where your cervix is. To do this you need to insert a finger inside the vagina so that the fingertip can feel the spongy bump at the top which is the cervix (very few women's cervixes are so far up the vagina that they can't be reached with the forefinger). Next, squeeze a 2-inch (5cm) length of spermicide cream inside the cap or diaphragm and smear it carefully around the inner rim; then do the same to the outer rim. Prepared with its spermicide, the springy rim is then squeezed between finger and thumb so that it forms a tube shape. It is then pushed gently into the vagina, where it will spring back to its original shape. You should be able to feel the bulge of the cervix through the rubber dome. The rim should sit neatly against the back wall of the vagina and the pubic bone at the front (you can feel this as a hard bump along the front wall of the vagina). The muscles of the wall of the vagina will hold it in place.

A cap or diaphragm can be put in place up to three hours before lovemaking but it shouldn't be removed sooner than six hours afterwards. In fact it can safely be left in place for up to 24 hours but you will need to apply more spermicide if you make love again during that time. Carefully used, a cap or diaphragm lasts for several years.

Health risks and the cap or diaphragm

Caps and diaphragms have virtually no harmful side-effects. Some users may find they are more prone to cystitis, or inflammation of the urinary tract and bladder (possibly caused by the rim pressing on the opening of the bladder), but this can be alleviated by switching to a softer-rimmed diaphragm or to the smaller cap. There's no need to worry about the effects of spermicide swallowed during oral sex: it may not be the greatest flavour ever invented but it is completely harmless.

CAPS AND DIAPHRAGMS — USED WITH A SPERMICIDE — COME IN SEVERAL SHAPES AND SIZES; CAREFUL FITTING IS ESSENTIAL WITH EVERY TYPE.

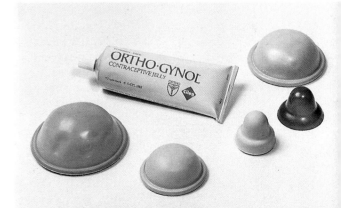

The Sponge

The newest addition to the range of barrier methods is the contraceptive sponge. Not all family planning clinics supply it, but it can be bought 'over the counter' without a prescription, though it is a little more expensive than other methods. The sponge looks like a large white marshmallow — about 2 in (5cm) across and nearly 1 in (2 cm) thick — with a dimple on one side which fits over the cervix, and a ribbon on the other side which makes it easy to pull out after use.

The sponge is pre-soaked with spermicide which is activated by moistening the sponge with a teaspoon or so of water and squeezing it once, gently. The function of the sponge is, in fact, mainly spermicidal; its effectiveness as a physical barrier is thought to be secondary.

How to use the sponge

Although the sponge does not need initial fitting by a doctor or nurse, as the cap or diaphragm does, it must be placed carefully over the cervix. You should ask your own doctor or local family planning clinic to show you how to insert it correctly. The big advantage of the sponge is that it can be left in place for up to 30 hours, and during that time you can make love as often as you like. Because it can be inserted up to 24 hours before lovemaking, and needs no additional spermicide, the sponge is less awkward and less messy than the diaphragm or cap. It should not be removed until at least six hours after last making love. It is not re-usable.

The big drawback of the sponge is its high failure rate, though this may improve as manufacturers perfect the method, but studies so far have shown that 15-20 out of 100 women using it can expect to get pregnant in any one year. Used on its own, the sponge is not very reliable, unless of course you don't really mind if you do get pregnant.

THE CONTRACEPTIVE SPONGE: EASY TO USE AND DESIGNED ATTRACTIVELY, BUT NOT THE SAFEST METHOD OF AVOIDING PREGNANCY.

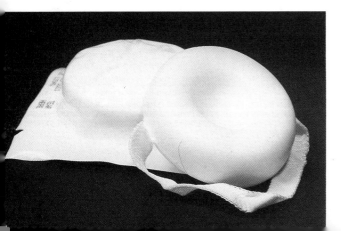

Natural family planning

Once regarded as a hit-or-miss method of birth control, natural family planning has been winning back favour in recent times, perhaps because it fits in better with a 'brown bread and muesli' lifestyle than the high-tech pill. Another thing in favour of natural methods is that they are 'couple' methods, requiring commitment from both partners. Even so, natural methods require expert counselling if they're to work, and they place a fairly hefty burden of responsibility and vigilance on the part of users. We do not supply sufficient information here. You must go to your doctor or family planning clinic for expert advice before trying any of these methods.

All natural family planning methods work by identifying the days of peak fertility in the menstrual cycle, and then by avoiding intercourse on these days. Most women are most likely to get pregnant *12 to 16 days before the first day of their period*, but because sperm can live for up to five days inside a woman's body, and an egg for up to two, the danger period for unprotected sex is rather longer than this.

The *temperature method* involves plotting changes which take place in the body temperature through the monthly cycle. The temperature of the body drops a little before ovulation and rises immediately afterwards. Temperature readings have to be taken every morning, using a thermometer specially designed to show small changes, and are marked up on a chart. After three days of recording a higher temperature reading, you can consider it safe to have sex. Because the body temperature changes with illness or when painkillers like aspirin are taken, ups and downs may not always be charted accurately.

The *Billings method*, also known as the *mucus method*, is based on detecting changes in the mucus around the cervix at different times of the month. Just before ovulation, the vagina and cervix become wetter and more slippery so that sperm can make their way up to the womb more easily. After ovulation, the cervix returns to its drier state and after at least four 'dry' days, it's safe to have sex again. For anyone with an active sex life, though, the presence of semen and naturally increased lubrication in the vagina can make it difficult to detect mucus changes.

The *calendar method*, in which 'safe' times for intercourse are judged on the basis of a whole year's monthly cycles, is no longer recognized as a method of natural family planning if no other protection is used. It is less reliable in women whose periods are not as regular as clockwork. Obviously, using a combination of natural family planning methods decrease the risk of pregnancy. Usually the mucus method *and* the temperature method are used together to pinpoint the fertile days of the month more exactly. Birth control experts call this the *sympto-thermal method.*

Health risks and natural methods?

As far as any meddling with the body is concerned, natural family planning methods can boast a clean record. But having to limit sex to those days on which pregnancy is not possible can put strains on a relationship, and to make it work, both partners have to share a commitment to the method.

NATURAL FAMILY PLANNING METHODS DEMAND COMMITMENT FROM BOTH PARTNERS — AND EXPERT ADVICE FROM YOUR DOCTOR OR FAMILY PLANNING CLINIC.

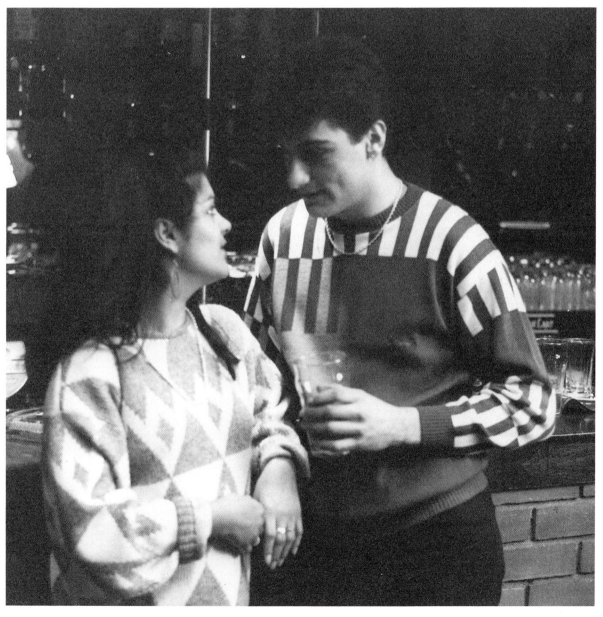

Other methods

For one reason or another, the following methods have definite drawbacks for young, single people and are so described in less detail.

Intra-uterine Device (IUD)

More commonly known as the coil or loop, an IUD is a small flexible device — usually made of plastic wound with copper — which sits inside the womb. It changes the lining of the womb in a way which makes it difficult for a fertilized egg to settle and grow. If you believe that life begins at the instant of conception you may have moral qualms about this method, because although it stops the egg developing, it doesn't stop it being fertilized. It doesn't interfere with lovemaking and for most of the time it can be more or less forgotten about. However, doctors do not consider IUDs a suitable choice for young women because of the increased risk of infection leading to infertility.

An IUD is always fitted by someone who is medically qualified — your own doctor, or family planning doctor or nurse. The device itself is squashed into an applicator tube like a drinking straw and passed through the narrow opening of the cervix. Once inside the womb, it opens out and regains its unsquashed shape. Because the cervix has to be stretched slightly to allow passage of the applicator tube, there is almost always a sharp twinge of pain during fitting. The pain is more noticeable if you are tense, but if you have never had a baby the muscles of both cervix and womb are quite tight, making it difficult to relax them. For this reason, many doctors prefer to fit an IUD during a period when the tissues are looser and softer, and also when there is no chance of a pregnancy already being under way.

The threads or tails of the IUD hang down into the vagina, and can easily be felt with a finger. Because the womb is capable of pushing out the IUD, these threads should be checked after each period to make sure the IUD is still in place. IUDs should be checked by a doctor three months after being fitted and then every year. Those wound with copper wire are usually replaced every two years to five years, though other types can be left longer than this without losing their effectiveness.

Because the threads of the IUD provide a direct route up into the womb for any germs present in the vagina, there is an extra risk of infection with this method. One of the reasons the IUD is not normally recommended to young women is that pelvic infection can lead to infertility. Also, women with a variety of sexual partners run a higher risk of infection, and would be better advised to use a different method.

Some women find they lose quite a lot of blood after having an IUD fitted, and that their periods are heavier, longer and sometimes more painful. These problems usually clear up after two or three periods, but they can be offputting.

The most common complaint couples have when making love protected by an IUD is that the tail or threads can be felt during intercourse. These usually soften after being soaked for a while in vaginal fluids, and coil themselves unobtrusively around the cervix, but occasionally they have to be trimmed back to avoid causing annoying sensations.

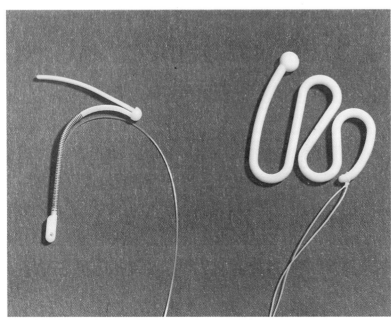

TWO POPULAR TYPES OF INTRA-UTERINE DEVICE (IUD): THE LIPPES LOOP (RIGHT) AND THE COPPER 7 (BOTH SHOWN LARGER THAN ACTUAL SIZE).

Withdrawal

Probably the oldest method of birth control, withdrawal is also the least effective. The best that can be said for it is that it is better than nothing, but not much.

Withdrawal is unsatisfactory for a number of reasons. The man has to pull his penis out of the woman's vagina a split second before he ejaculates, which means that he has to have absolute self-control and she has to have nerves of steel. Even if he does manage to be quick enough off the mark, a small amount of semen — enough to cause a pregnancy — may already have leaked from his penis before ejaculation. Not only is withdrawal not very reliable, it is also not very satisfying. The sudden jolt of the man's body away from his partner's at such a tender moment is unlikely to enhance their lovemaking. So withdrawal is best reserved for ill-timed emergencies when absolutely nothing else is available.

Injectables

These work hormonally, like the progestogen-only pill, but instead of taking a daily pill, you have one injection which effectively prevents conception for eight to twelve weeks (depending on the injectable used). The hormone in the injection is released slowly over that period, preventing ovulation. One of the criticisms of injectables is that they often disrupt the menstrual cycle, causing heavy bleeding or an absence of periods altogether. There have also been scares about injectables increasing the risk of cancer of the cervix (see page 185) but the evidence is complex and contradictory. Injectables are not recommended for younger women unless they find it impossible to remember to take the pill every day or unless, for medical reasons, a pregnancy would be fatal. Injectables can only be prescribed by a doctor.

Spermicides

Used alone, spermicides are a fairly bad bet in terms of preventing pregnancy. The chemicals which put sperm out of action come in the form of jellies, creams, foams and pessaries (small tablets which dissolve in the vagina). Though they are all best used with another method (such as the sheath, cap or diaphragm), foams and pessaries are probably the most effective on their own. Spermicidal foams must be injected into the vagina using the special applicator no more than half an hour before lovemaking, and shouldn't be washed out by taking a bath for at least eight hours afterwards. Pessaries need to be pushed deep into the vagina at least ten minutes before lovemaking to make sure they dissolve in time, and they cannot be considered effective for longer than an hour. In the case of a sheath bursting or slipping off, a quick application of foam might help to head off disaster. The truth is that spermicidal applications *after* unprotected sex are a most unreliable way of preventing pregnancy, though they may offer temporary psychological comfort.

'Morning-after' birth control

Strictly for emergencies. If you've had sex without using any method of birth control, or if a sheath fails, there are two eleventh-hour methods of preventing pregnancy. Neither is strictly 'morning after' in the literal sense, but you have to act fast.

The morning-after pill consists of two doses of a specially high-strength version of the combined pill; *one must be taken within three days (72 hours) of* unprotected sex, and *the other 12 hours after the first*. You can get these from your own doctor or family planning doctor but you must tell them how urgent it is. Side-effects are likely to be more pronounced: you may feel or be sick, suffer irregular heavy bleeding and headaches. These are not harmful but they may be unpleasant. This method should *not* be used regularly.

The second method involves having an IUD fitted within five days of unprotected sex (see page 78). A doctor must fit the device and again it's essential that you manage to get across the sense of urgency. The egg may already have been fertilized but the IUD will stop it implanting in the womb. If you think this method of birth control is suitable for you, the IUD can be left in place.

Sterilization

Sterilization of both men and women is performed by a doctor who cuts or blocks the tubes which carry the eggs in women and the sperm in men. A large number of couples — as many as one in five in Britain on current estimates — eventually settle for this method once they are sure they have had all the children they want.

But until someone comes up with techniques that are guaranteed reversible, sterilization cannot really be recommended for young couples. There are too many unknown factors. Will you *always* dread the patter of tiny feet? Will you *always* be with your current partner? If not, will your next partner share your views about not having children? For these reasons, most doctors are extremely reluctant to go ahead with the operation with those who are single, unmarried or childless. If you're absolutely determined, you may get somewhere, but the counselling process usually weeds out all except those who are hell-bent on not becoming parents.

Coping with an unplanned pregnancy___

If you've had unprotected intercourse, or if a birth control method has failed for some reason, it's the easiest thing in the world to find yourself pregnant. A suspicion that this might have happened can throw you into a turmoil of anxiety and confusion.

One common coping pattern is to ignore the symptoms or cling to the hope that they'll go away, like a bad cold. Understandable though this reaction is, it's the worst possible one in terms of seeking help. If you decide to go ahead and have the baby, the sooner you book in with your doctor for antenatal care, the better the chances of a healthy pregnancy and a healthy baby. And if you decide to end the pregnancy, a termination is far safer and easier if it is carried out early in the pregnancy rather than later.

Am I pregnant?

If you suspect you are pregnant, the first step is to find out if you really are. The first sign of pregnancy is, of course, a missed period. But often within a couple of weeks of this other signs begin to appear. Breasts feel fuller and sometimes the nipples feel tingly and sensitive; you may feel sick and need to urinate more often.

The only way to find out for sure whether these are real or imaginary symptoms is to have a pregnancy test. Your doctor will carry this out without charge, and pregnancy advisory services (listed at the back of the book) will do the same for a small fee. Either way, you'll need to take along an early-morning sample of urine in a clean container. Alternatively, you can do the test yourself using one of the commercial packs obtainable from chemists (ask for a pregnancy testing kit). These tests are easy to use and can be as reliable as those carried out professionally, provided you follow the instructions. Pregnancy tests should not be carried out until at least 14 days after the first day your period was due, or you may get a misleading result. If the test shows up as negative, you can first thank your lucky stars and *then* read carefully through this chapter to avoid another 'scare'. Just occasionally, however, the result of a test can be wrong. So if you still haven't had your period after another two weeks, have another test. If the result is still negative, you're in the clear.

What if the test is positive

You have some important decision-making to do *quickly*. Whether you decide to go ahead and have the baby will depend very much on your circumstances. Do you have a stable relationship? What is your housing and financial situation? What are you planning on doing with your life? It also depends on your moral stand on the abortion issue. People generally tend to divide up into those who believe that every woman should have the right to choose when and whether she has a baby and not be penalized for contraceptive failure or thoughtlessness, and those who believe in the right to life of the unborn child and see abortion as amounting to murder.

As with many other controversial issues, we may hold very strong views on the subject until we're personally involved, and then we may start to feel very differently. A woman who has previously been a fierce defender of the rights of the unborn child may find herself wavering when her own life is in danger of disruption. Contrariwise, the stalwart supporter of abortion on demand may feel differently when a baby is growing inside her own body.

Because of these difficult and complicated feelings, the importance of good counselling cannot be over-stressed. Whether you're leaning towards continuing the pregnancy or terminating it, you'll need expert help. Several organizations offer counselling services and give practical help. Others offer advice and information on pregnancy and childbirth. Again, their addresses can be found at the end of the book. Men should not be excluded from counselling, so remember to include your partner if possible.

If you decide to have the baby, you should see your doctor as soon as possible to arrange good antenatal care. If you decide not to, you can have an abortion provided that your case meets the grounds laid down legally. Abortion has been legal in England, Wales and Scotland since 1967, but in Northern Ireland and the Isle of Man the operation is still illegal except on very restricted medical grounds.

In order to carry out an abortion, two doctors must be satisfied that one or more of the following conditions applies to you.

Would you be more careful if it was you that got pregnant?

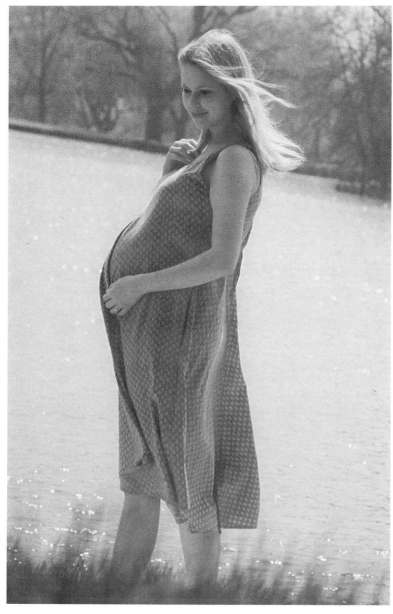

■ There would be greater risk to your life if the pregnancy continued, than if it were terminated.

■ There would be greater risk to your mental and physical health if the pregnancy continued, than if it were terminated.

■ There would be greater risk to the physical and mental health of existing children if the pregnancy continued, than if it were terminated.

■ There is reason to suspect that the child might be born mentally or physically handicapped.

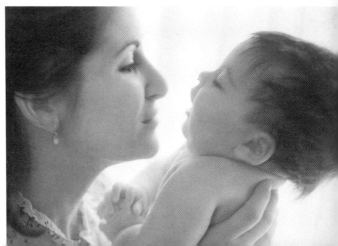

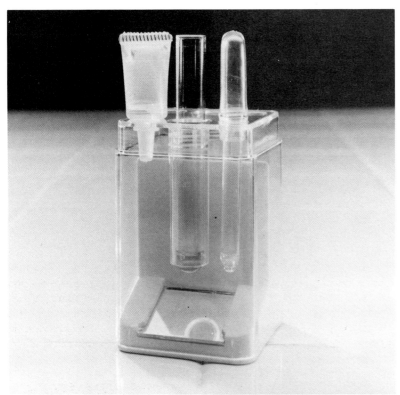

HOME PREGNANCY TESTING KITS CAN
BE BOUGHT FROM ANY CHEMISTS
AND ARE SIMPLE TO USE.

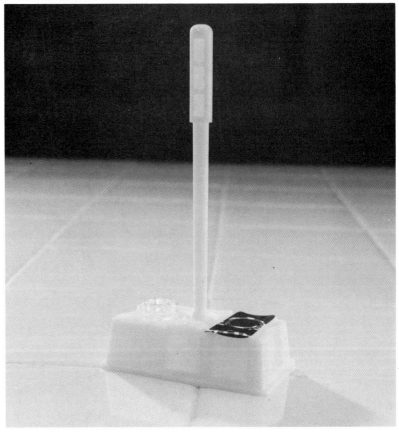

The second condition tends to apply to young women more than the others; the 'risk to mental health' often being the deciding factor. In theory, provided these conditions have been met, abortion is carried out free through the National Health Service. In practice, provision for the operation varies greatly from one part of the country to another. There are charitable organizations who provide the operation for a relatively small cost and some commercial organizations who cash in on human misfortune and charge the earth. Only the former are listed at the end of the book.

What does abortion involve?
Abortion is a safe and simple operation provided it is carried out in the early stages of pregnancy. During the very early weeks of pregnancy (though not earlier than six) a process known as vacuum aspiration can be carried out — the contents of the womb, including the fertilized egg, are removed by suction. After the twelfth week of pregnancy an operation called a 'D and C' (Dilatation and Curettage) is carried out — the entrance to the womb is dilated and the contents 'scraped' out (this sounds more savage than it is; the instrument is in fact more like a spatula than a knife). Abortions later in pregnancy closely resemble actual births and involve the use of artificial hormones which mimic the natural ones which start up the contractions which expel the baby from the womb at birth. After 24 weeks of pregnancy, a foetus is deemed capable of independent life, which means that it could live outside the mother's body, and so no abortions are undertaken after this time. In fact at this late stage abortion would be much less safe, and could be far more upsetting for the mother, than carrying the baby to term.

All these methods of abortion usually require a general anaesthetic and an overnight stop in a clinic or hospital, though whether this is insisted upon will depend very much on local circumstances, and on how advanced the pregnancy is.

Abortion after-care
In addition to counselling before abortion, some women find they need help and advice after abortion to help them come to terms with feelings of loss and possibly guilt. This may take the form of joining a self-help group or seeing a trained counsellor or therapist (see list of useful addresses page 186). No woman should be afraid to seek help with difficult feelings after an abortion.

COUNSELLING BOTH BEFORE AND AFTER ABORTION ARE EQUALLY IMPORTANT TO COPE WITH EMOTIONAL DIFFICULTIES.

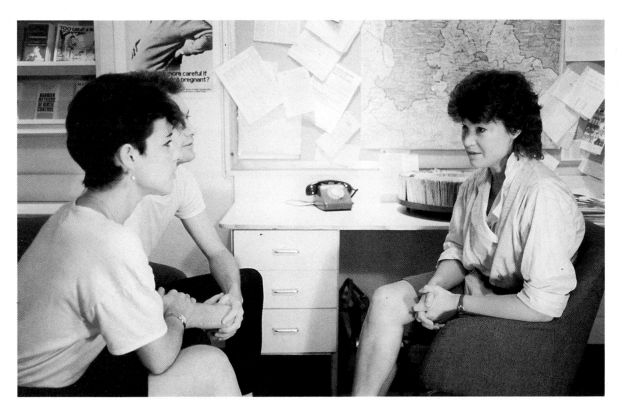

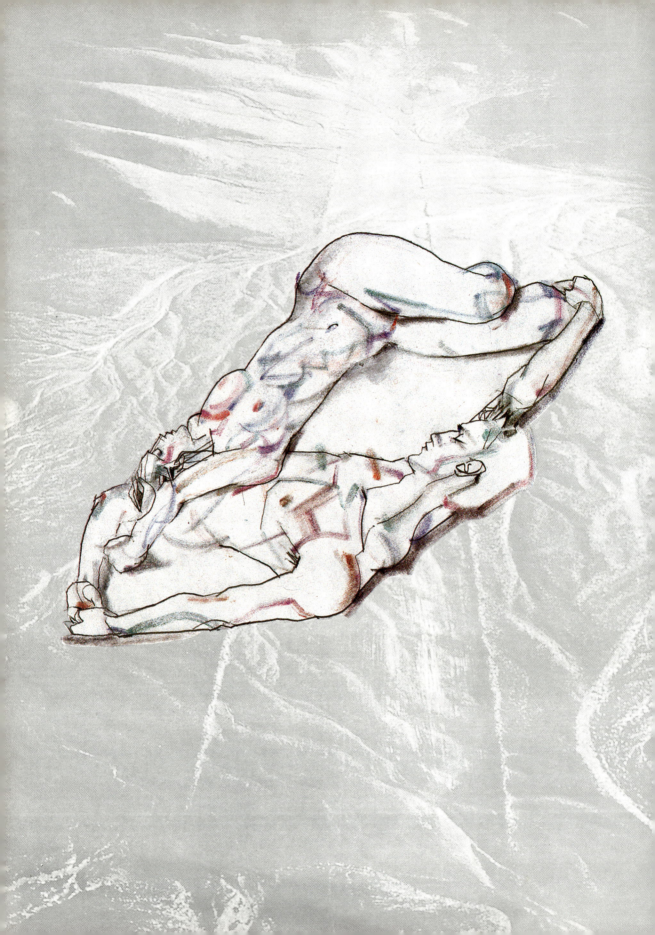

6
Knowing your body

A central belief of this book is that sex is at least 50 per cent emotions and feelings, and probably a good deal more. But that doesn't mean we can totally forget about bodies. Nor does it mean we need only know about the part they play in producing babies, the reproductive plumbing of sex. Sex is about pleasure as well as procreation and our bodies are designed to provide us with enjoyment as well as offspring.

Even today there is still a great deal of ignorance about the physical side of sex. Sexual ignorance can lead to very real problems, but it can also give rise to fears and anxieties which can inhibit pleasure. There must be countless men and women who have shared a lifetime of sex without ever being really familiar with the intimate parts of each other's bodies. Learning by discovery is fun, but a little knowledge helps.

This chapter doesn't aim to make you an expert in physiology but it does aim to give you a basic grounding in sexual anatomy. Being familiar with your sex organs helps you to accept yourself as you are and others as they are. It's important to like yourself without your clothes on — it's part of liking yourself generally — though it can be difficult, in the cold light of day, for a man to believe that the wrinkly limp bit of skin between his legs is beautiful, or for a woman to accept that the slippery pink folds between hers are beautiful too. Yet to someone physically close to us, our intimate parts *are* beautiful, and the sincerest statement of this is for our partner to want to look at and touch them.

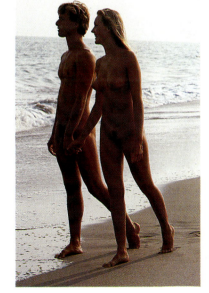

It is often said that the largest of all our sex organs is the brain — it masterminds all our physical responses, spins amazing fantasies, and is always on the alert for the sexual potential in a voice, a gesture, a swing of the hips…But the emphasis in these chapters is on 'primary' sex organs[*], those parts of the body most directly involved in intercourse. Those areas of the body which make us feel sexually aroused when they're touched, kissed or stroked are called erogenous zones — in this sense the whole surface of the body is potentially an erogenous zone since every inch of our skin can respond with the right partner. Men, more than women, have a tendency to home in on the genital area, but if all-over stimulation is on offer men like it just as much as women! One of the biggest sexual favours you can exchange with a partner is to gently and slowly explore each other's bodies. You can do this with your hands and fingers, or with your mouth, lips, tongue, and so on. And you can get just as much pleasure from stimulating your lover's body as you do from the sensations of your own.

[*]The more familiar names by which these are known cannot be guaranteed not to give offence in print, so we've used the more medical and scientific ones. You can substitute those you feel more comfortable with.

Male sex organs

Since men's sex organs are, for the most part, more visible than women's, they are generally less cloaked in mystery. This can be both an advantage and a disadvantage. Penises have an annoying habit of becoming erect at the wrong time and refusing to do so at the right time. They also cause their owners a great deal of anxiety because of their shape or their size (see page 122). There's no guarantee you'll recognize yours among the drawings (to show the full range we'd need to draw thousands of specimens!) but you'll get some idea of the diversity which passes for normal.

Normally a man's penis hangs limply downwards, but in its erect state it points horizontally outwards or slightly upwards at an angle. Three spongy cylinders make up its length and, when a man is sexually excited, blood is pumped into their hollow cavities and the penis becomes longer and firmer. Contrary to popular belief, a penis has no muscles along its length, nor any bone, just a ring of muscle around the base which tightens during sexual excitement and helps to keep it erect. Down the centre of the penis runs the *urethra*, a narrow tube which performs the dual function of carrying urine from the bladder and semen from the *vas deferens* (the tube which leads from the testes). But it never does *both* at the same time. During erection, a small muscle closes off the entrance to the bladder so that no urine can be passed.

Outwardly the penis is made up of a stem or *shaft* and a head or *glans*, which together resemble a long-stalked mushroom. The shaft is covered with loose, wrinkly, darkish skin which, in uncircumcised men, extends over the tip to form the foreskin. As the penis swells during erection, this skin becomes tighter and the wrinkles smooth out. At the same time, it pulls back slightly from the tip of the penis leaving the plum-like head exposed.

The head is studded with a mass of nerve endings which make it the most sensitive part of the penis. The whole of the rim or *ridge* (where the head joins the shaft) is capable of providing some very pleasant sensations, but on the underside is an exquisitely sensitive area, the *frenum*, which looks rather like a taut bowstring. the lightest touch applied to this part of the penis is enough to produce an erection, and if sustained for any length of time is likely to lead to orgasm.

Below and behind the penis is a pouch of slightly coarser, slightly hairy skin called the *scrotal sac* or *scrotum* which houses the *testes*. The testes produce sperm and *testosterone*, the hormone responsible for the male sex drive. Each testis contains about half a mile of threadlike tubing which transports the sperm-laden *semen* to its vas deferens. And every teaspoonful of semen ejaculated teems with more than 300,000,000 sperm — Nature takes massive precautions to ensure that at least one sperm reaches the egg!

Because sperm are destroyed by temperatures higher than blood heat the scrotal sac normally hangs down away from the body where it is cooler. During fear, extreme cold or sexual excitement, the testes contract, become harder and more compact, and draw up to fit snugly against the body. In its loose, descended state, the skin of the scrotum is less sensitive to touch; contracted, it becomes very sensitive to *light* caresses (the testes are so tender that even a little over-enthusiastic pressure can be painful enough to banish erotic sensations altogether).

Behind the testes and in front of the *anus* is a small flat area, the *perineum*. This is an often neglected pleasure zone and has great potential, as does the anus in many men, for arousal.

FAR LEFT: AN UNCIRCUMCISED PENIS.
LEFT: A CIRCUMCISED PENIS.

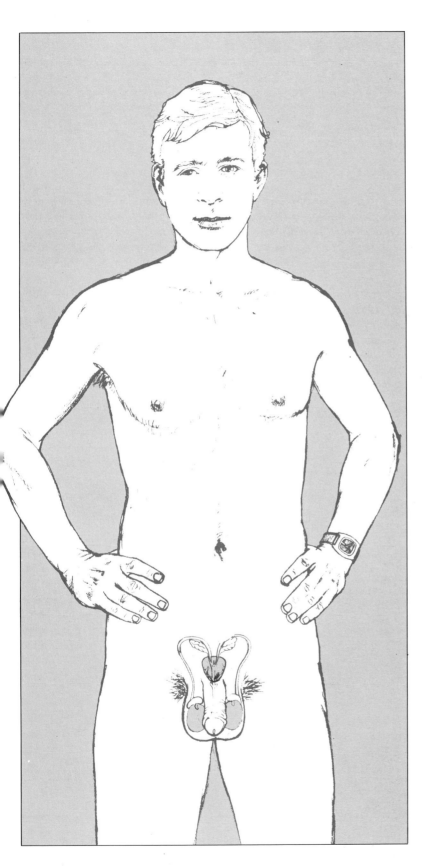

THE MALE SEX ORGANS. A PENIS HAS
NO MUSCLES ALONG ITS LENGTH —
NOR ANY BONE — JUST A RING OF
MUSCLE AROUND THE BASE WHICH
TIGHTENS DURING SEXUAL
EXCITEMENT AND HELPS TO KEEP IT
ERECT. SPERM DO NOT THRIVE AT
BODY TEMPERATURE, WHICH IS WHY
THEY ARE STORED IN THE EXTERNAL
TESTICLES.

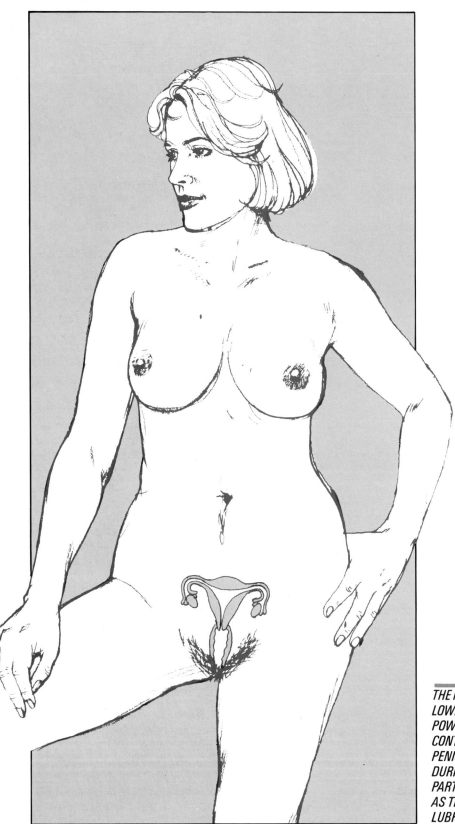

THE FEMALE SEX ORGANS. THE
LOWER PART OF THE VAGINA HAS
POWERFUL MUSCLES WHICH CAN
CONTRACT AROUND THE MAN'S
PENIS DURING INTERCOURSE. ALSO
DURING INTERCOURSE, THE OUTER
PART OF THE VAGINA BECOMES MOIST
AS THE WALLS SECRETE THEIR
LUBRICATING FLUIDS.

Female sex organs

Legs together, there is little to see of a woman's sex organs except a neat fleshy triangle at the base of her tummy; this is the *pubic mound* or 'mound of Venus'. From puberty onwards, this is covered by crisp, curly hair which in some women grows up towards the navel. Beneath the pubic mound are two large fleshy folds of skin, the *labia majora*. Most of the time these lie close together, but when they are parted, two thinner, more delicate folds beneath — the *labia minora* — can be seen. When a woman is sexually excited, these swell slightly and darken to a deeper shade of pink.

Nestling between the inner folds of the *vulva*, the name given to a woman's outer sex organs, is a tiny organ, the *clitoris*, which can be found by wiggling a finger forwards until a tiny bump is found. Small though it may be, the clitoris is in fact the powerhouse of a woman's sexual feelings. Though there are still men who operate under the illusion that the vagina is the centre of a woman's sexual pleasure, it is now established beyond any shadow of doubt that the clitoris is the focus of her most intense sensations. And if there are any remaining doubts about whether nice girls are supposed to enjoy sex, or just put up with it in order to have babies, the existence of the clitoris knocks them firmly on the head. It plays no part at all in reproduction except to make sex play more pleasurable.

Physically, the clitoris resembles a small penis, complete with a diminutive shaft and head. In terms of nerve endings per unit length, it is probably even more sensitive than the penis and so spends most of its life protected by a small hood or sleeve of tissue. Like the penis, the clitoris is made up of spongy tissue which, during sexual arousal, is engorged by blood and becomes fuller and firmer. When this happens the hood pulls back and exposes the delicate tip, but at the peak of excitement it shrinks back into its hood again.

The clitoris can be stimulated directly by stroking the shaft slowly and gently to begin with and then faster and with a firmer touch as excitement mounts. (The head is far too sensitive in most women for direct touching at the start of sex.) To reach orgasm most women need sustained and uninterrupted stimulation of the clitoris. During intercourse the pressure of the man's pubic bone against the clitoris may be sufficient stimulation for some women. For others the tugging action of the penis on the whole vulval area does the trick. But a large proportion of women, maybe the majority, need direct and continuous stimulation of the clitoris by hand (either partner can provide it), at the same time as penetration, in order to reach orgasm.

Moving down from the clitoris, you come to a small opening, the *urethra*, which leads from the bladder, and then to a larger opening, the *vagina*. In virgins, the entrance to the vagina is partly covered by a thin membrane of skin, the *hymen*, but never completely since a gap is always needed to allow menstrual blood to seep away. A great deal of importance used to be attached (and still is in some parts of the world) to the girl being able to prove that her hymen was in one piece on her wedding night. In fact, very few women make it to first intercourse without their hymen showing some signs of wear and tear — through using tampons, sporting activity, masturbation, or whatever — and few men today would turn a hair if they found their lover was not 'virgo intacta'.

The vagina itself is about 3 in (7.5 cm) long and extremely elastic, so much so that it can accommodate an erect penis double its length and several times its width, not to mention a baby's head at birth. The lower part of the vagina has powerful muscles which can contract around the penis, producing pleasurable hugging sensations, and its walls secrete a milky, mucus fluid which lubricates the vagina. Only this outer part of the vagina has enough nerve endings in it to allow very much sensation in most women.

At its upper end, the vagina opens out into a wider section which billows out like a balloon during sexual arousal. Here there are fewer nerve endings and therefore less sensation, though a minority of women report that the neck of the womb or *cervix* is sensitive to touch. If you slide a finger full length into the vagina, this can be felt as a slippery bump at the top, with a dimple in the middle. Note that a man's penis cannot penetrate the womb. Entry is restricted to a tiny opening in the cervix through which menstrual blood can flow downwards and sperm can swim upwards. A man may *feel* as if his penis is entering the womb, and it may be a highly exciting thought, but he is more likely to have felt it slide into the groove around the cervix.

No discussion of female pleasure spots would be complete without a mention of the *G spot*. This is a specially sensitive zone thought to lie about 1 in (2.5cm) inside the vagina on its front wall, which, it is claimed, can trigger orgasm and even lead to female ejaculation. The comparatively recent discovery of its possible existence has made G spot-searching a fashionable sexual pastime! Women who *do* find they're blessed with such a spot should count themselves lucky because scientific evidence for its existence is very shaky.

As with men, the *perineum* and *anus* are generally neglected areas of a woman's body, perhaps because our early childhood training teaches us that these regions are somehow 'dirty' and not to be touched. With careful personal hygiene there is no reason why they should not be touched, and few women fail to respond if a finger is traced lightly around the anus and along the flat muscular patch of skin in front of it.

A woman's *breasts*, though they may not be thought of as primary sex organs, are an important source of pleasure for both sexes. Most men are quickly turned on by the sight of a shapely bosom and most women enjoy having their breasts and nipples stroked or kissed. A minority can even reach orgasm as a result of nipple stimulation. Whether breasts are large or small makes absolutely no difference to the pleasure they give their owner. Only if she feels self-conscious about being over- or under-endowed might size affect enjoyment (see page 123).

During sexual arousal, many women's breasts show some physical changes. They may plump up slightly and develop a pink-tinged rash. At the peak of excitement the nipples often stand erect and many men knowingly look for this as an acid test that their partner has 'come'. Because different people react in different ways, this cannot be taken as a cast-iron guarantee! Erect nipples do generally show that a woman is highly aroused, but non-erect nipples do not infallibly mean that she isn't.

What happens to your body when you are sexually excited?

First, a word of warning. Many books on sex deal with this topic under headings like 'Arousal Patterns' or 'Sexual Response', as if there were a standard way of reacting that applied to everyone. They usually draw heavily on the work of sexologists who have charted many different people's sexual responses and summarized them as peaks and troughs and plateaux in graphs.

One problem with this approach is that it suggests there is a 'correct' way of responding, when in fact sexual response differs from person to person and from one occasion to the next in the same person. Many people's sexual responses *don't* fit neatly into those charted by experts.

Another problem with seeing sexual response as a neat progression up through levels of excitement is that it implies the whole thing is plain sailing. You set off on your sexual voyage and on you go without stopping until you reach the Holy Grail of orgasm. If you're not seeing stars by the end of the trip you think your navigational skills are at fault.

Sex is rarely like that. Sometimes it might be, but just as often there'll be times when you drift into daydreams, when you stop to admire the scenery, or when you're frankly bored or not in the mood.

Lovers should give themselves and one another permission to take a breather and have a cuddle, to enjoy the feelings as and when they come. It is, after all, very nice to be physically close to someone whether you're pulsating and palpitating or not.

So why bother to describe 'sexual response' at all? For two fairly good reasons. The first is that the strong physical sensations that are a part of intercourse can be quite unnerving if you're caught unawares. Knowing that what is happening is normal can be reassuring. Secondly, knowing something about the reactions of your partner can help you to adapt the pace of your lovemaking to suit you both.

So read on by all means, but be wary of taking it all too literally. If you start taking mental meter readings of your own and each other's excitement levels, there's a danger you'll switch off altogether.

If you're a woman...

The obvious difference between men and women is that women generally take far longer than men to become fully excited. But many of the signs of excitement are the same for both sexes. Breathing quickens, the heart beat gets faster, muscles tighten in various parts of the body and there's a warm flush of pleasure as blood flow to the body increases.

At the same time, changes are taking place in the sex organs. As blood flows into it, the whole area of the vulva becomes firm and swollen and deepens in colour, often to a dark shade of pink. The outer part of the vagina widens and becomes moist as the walls secrete their lubricating fluids or 'love juices', and these may seep out to make the outer area wet too. This reaction happens quite quickly and ensures that the penis can push easily into the vagina, but it should *not* be taken as a sign that a woman is ready for this to happen.

The clitoris now becomes larger and firmer, and emerges from its hood, which makes it easier to stimulate. What was previously a vaguely felt bump now becomes a recognizable shape and the cylindrical shaft can easily be felt.

The breasts too show changes. They may swell slightly and develop a rosy flush, and the nipples may stand out and become erect.

As excitement increases, the inner part of the vagina continues to balloon out, but the outer part narrows as its walls swell to hold the penis more snugly. At this stage the whole of the vulva is likely to be extremely sensitive. Many women tremble, as the muscles of the body jerk and twitch involuntarily. At this stage, orgasm is usually close but partners who know each other well often prefer to prolong this as the most pleasurable phase of their lovemaking.

At a certain point, either as a result of her partner touching or rubbing her clitoris or other parts of her vulva, or as he moves his penis inside her, a woman may get a feeling of losing control — often felt as 'going over the top'. The feeling of having reached a point of no return may come on several seconds before orgasm and many women describe it as even more pleasurable than the actual moment of climax. When this happens, there's likely to be a sudden warm glow starting in the solar plexus (in the pit of the stomach) which radiates out to all parts of the body. A series of short rhythmical contractions begins in the vagina and may spread to the womb and even to the whole body. The muscles in many parts of the body may go into a kind of involuntary spasm, including those of the face, which can take on an anguished expression.

Just before orgasm, breath is normally drawn in sharply so that at the moment of release there is characteristically a cry or sigh. This may be a barely audible whimper or moan, or it may be let out more dramatically as a shriek or scream. The noise level doesn't necessarily have anything to do with the enjoyment level!

Women are generally capable of reaching more than one climax more easily than men *More* doesn't necessarily mean *better* in sexual matters, but if a woman is not fully satisfied by one orgasm, it may be better for a couple to adjust their routine so that she can come more than once before her partner does.

After orgasm, the body quickly settles back to normal. Muscles relax, blood flow returns to normal, and the sex organs return to their usual colour, size, shape and position. (This also happens when orgasm has not occurred but it takes rather longer.) At the same time there's a feeling of relaxation, wellbeing, contentment, a sense of being very, very close.

WOMEN'S AROUSAL PATTERN

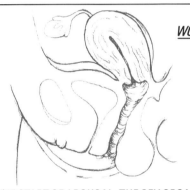

1. AT THE START OF AROUSAL: THE SEX ORGANS BECOME FULLER AND FIRMER, THE OUTER WALLS OF THE VAGINA WIDEN AND BECOME MORE MOIST.

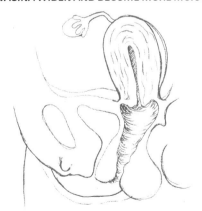

2. AS EXCITEMENT MOUNTS: THE OUTER PART OF THE VAGINA IS STILL EXPANDED AND THE WALLS OF THE INNER PART BALLOON OUT TOO.

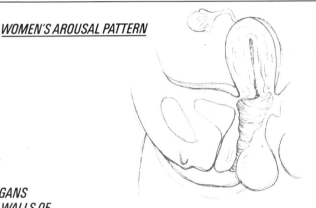

3. CLOSE TO ORGASM: THE OUTER PART OF THE VAGINA NARROWS, MUSCLE TENSION INCREASES UNTIL AND AT THE POINT OF CLIMAX THE VAGINA CONTRACTS RHYTHMICALLY.

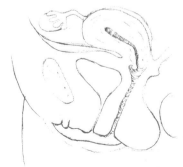

4. AFTER ORGASM, ALL SEXUAL ORGANS RELAX AND RETURN TO THEIR NORMAL POSITION.

If you're a man...

The first sign of sexual arousal in a man is usually that he has an erection. The source of excitement may be a picture in his mind — the sight of someone he finds sexually attractive, or a fantasy — or some form of physical contact. Either way, the effect is the same. Blood rushes to numerous parts of the body, including the penis, which becomes larger and firmer and alters the angle it makes with the body.

These changes take place along with other bodily changes similar to those which occur in a woman. A man's breathing and heart beat get faster, his nipples may become erect and the same sex flush may spread across the front of his body.

It's worth mentioning that all these changes are, at this stage, capable of going into reverse. If a man's mind wanders off, if the caresses he found stimulating are not kept up, or if the stimulation has been going on for a long time with no variation, he is capable of losing his erection, though it returns quickly when stimulation starts up again.

As excitement mounts, muscles tense in the legs and buttocks, and also in the face, which may take on a somewhat intense expression. The testes and scrotum harden and are drawn up tight against the body. As the moment of ejaculation gets closer, a man's pelvis often starts to thrust and a small amount of clear fluid may seep out from the head of the penis. Although the purpose of this fluid is probably to lubricate the penis, it often contains some sperm, which is why withdrawal (see page 79) is not a reliable form of birth control.

There are two fairly distinct steps to orgasm in a man. The first begins as semen travelling up from the testes pours into the urethra. As this happens, the urethra widens — an intensely pleasurable sensation. It is at this point, when he knows he is coming and that it's no longer possible to hold back, that excitement is at its peak. Moments later semen is forced out of the penis by the pumping action of the urethra, which contracts strongly four or five times. The semen may shoot out with some force or it may simply ooze out, depending partly on how long it is since ejaculation last happened.

The term 'ejaculation' is often used interchangeably with 'orgasm' in men, but correctly speaking it refers only to the moment when semen spurts out of the penis. As in women, orgasm itself is a total bodily experience of which ejaculation is only a part. The pleasurable feelings spread to all parts of the body.

Shortly after ejaculation (and sometimes immediately) the penis goes back to its normal size and the scrotum and testes settle back to their usual position. Muscular tension ebbs away and most men experience deep feelings of relaxation, even of drowsiness, at this point. Some, to their partner's disgust and annoyance, even want to go to sleep. A man is very lucky (and probably very young) if his penis springs back to life again very soon.

A common worry for men is that they will feel extreme discomfort and even some pain if they don't have an orgasm. Certainly muscle tension and the 'bursting' feeling caused by engorgement of blood in the sex organs are relieved faster after orgasm, but this happens anyway after a little while even if there has been no orgasm. Any discomfort is only temporary.

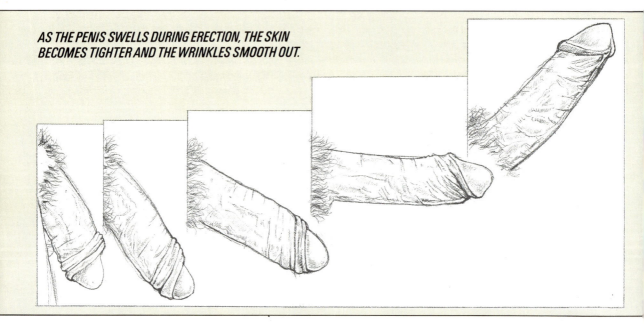

AS THE PENIS SWELLS DURING ERECTION, THE SKIN BECOMES TIGHTER AND THE WRINKLES SMOOTH OUT.

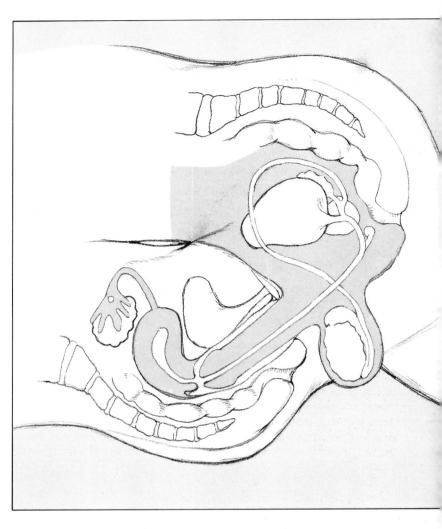

SEXUAL INTERCOURSE INVOLVES THE COMING TOGETHER AND SMOOTH COMBINATION OF TWO COMPLICATED BUT HIGHLY EFFICIENT PIECES OF MACHINERY — THE MALE AND FEMALE SEX ORGANS.

'What does it feel like to have an orgasm?'
Just in case all this sounds as if erections, lubrications and ejaculations are the only terms in which sex can be described, here are some real-life, warm-blooded human beings describing their orgasmic sensations.

'It's the building up of a good kind of tension, with the release of all this build-up in one great rush that makes your whole body tingle and feel very pleasurable. A weakening feeling, which is great. I just want to stay still for a long time.'

'It's intense excitement of the whole body. Vibrations in the stomach. Your mind can only consider your own desires at the moment of climax. After, you feel like you're floating — a sense of joyful tiredness.'

'It's a very pleasurable sensation. All my tensions have built up to a peak, and suddenly they're released. It feels like a great upheaval. Like all of the organs in the stomach area have turned over.'

'It's extremely pleasurable, but it can be so violent that the feeling of uncontrol is frightening. It's hard to describe because it's as if I'm in a kind of limbo, only conscious of release.'

'I often see spots in front of my eyes during orgasm. The feeling itself is so difficult to describe...it's the most pleasurable of all sensations. I suppose the words "fluttering sensation" describe the physical feelings I get. All my nerve endings sort of burst and quiver.'

'It's a building-up of tension, like getting ready for take-off from a launching pad. Then a sudden blossoming relief that extends all over the body.'

The elusive orgasm

The last hundred years have seen a sea of change in attitudes towards sexuality, particularly women's sexuality. From being expected to put up with sex rather than enjoy it, women now feel expected to produce orgasms to order, preferably multiple, simultaneously, noisily, and in places they didn't know were there. Failure to meet these exacting standards has been the cause of much anxiety in both women and men, yet *worrying* about *not* having an orgasm is one of the surest ways to block sensations.

'How can I tell whether I've had an orgasm?'

It's generally true to say that if you've experienced orgasm you know about it. But some people don't trust their own experience; they wonder instead if it matches up to that of their friends or to the earth-moving episodes they read about in books. Of one thing you can be sure: everyone responds differently and each orgasm can vary in intensity. For some,

orgasm may be a body-racking experience, complete with convulsive spasms; others may feel only a gentle genital ripple. Some let out ear-piercing yells; others just sigh or moan softly. The test of a good sexual experience is not what the machine clocks up, nor has it anything to do with the decibel level. Whether your sex ends with a whimper or a bang, the important thing is how you feel about yourself and about each other.

'How can I make my partner come?'

There are no magic formulae, no step-by-step routines, and no miracle techniques. Not experiencing orgasm may have something to do with technique, but it's just as likely to be the result of anxiety. One of the easiest ways to stop someone having an orgasm is to show him or her that the pressure is on. Stop trying so hard and you may find it happens naturally.

This said, there are two essentials to bear in mind. First, know what pleases you. Second, know how to

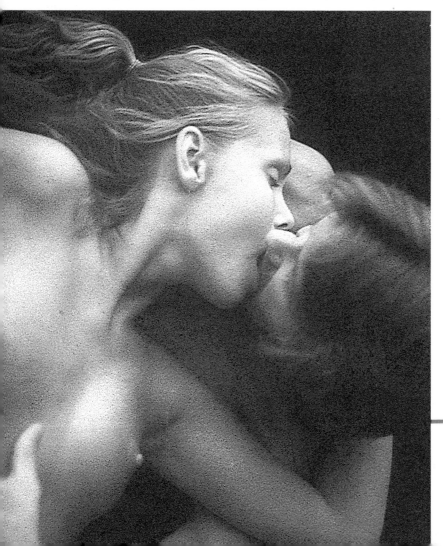

A GREAT DEAL OF SEXUAL PLEASURE COMES FROM BEING CLOSE TO ANOTHER WARM BODY. GIVING AND TAKING PLEASURE DOESN'T ALWAYS HAVE TO BE DURING INTERCOURSE.

convey this to your partner. You may find it helpful to look at the section on masturbation (page 124) and on talking about sex (page 110).

'If we can't come together, should we stay together?'

If there are feelings like this washing around in a relationship, they won't help to create a harmonious sex life. If one of you feels the other is saying 'Come or I'll go', you're not going to respond easily. At the moment of orgasm we're at our most vulnerable — all our defences are down. We're unlikely to let go completely with someone we can't trust our feelings to. Certainly a woman's orgasm is made easier by any conditions which make her feel that the man she is having sex with can be counted on to stay around afterwards. A perfect sex life takes time, careful nurturing, and absolute trust.

'Is it important to come at the same time?'

Many people believe that simultaneous orgasm represents the peak of sexual achievement. Others prefer to double their enjoyment by experiencing their own and their partner's climax separately. Some men find their sensations enhanced if they come just after their partner, when the rhythmical contractions of the vagina give their penis its final trigger. Other couples find the easiest time for a woman to come is after the man, when she no longer feels she's holding him up. Against the simultaneous orgasm, it must be said that it is difficult to concentrate on someone else's pleasure when you're losing control yourself!

There is no one pattern or tempo which is better than another. If you enjoy making love it doesn't matter a jot if it's not synchronized like clockwork.

'I've never had a multiple orgasm'

Some people have the capacity to come more than once in one lovemaking session, women more than men generally. But just because some *do* doesn't mean that everyone *should*. There's certainly no proof that enjoyment increases. Ten snacks a day is no more satisfying than two good meals!

'Do women have more than one type of orgasm?'

It used to be thought so. The theory was that clitoral orgasms were immature and unfeminine, and that well-adjusted, fully mature women only had vaginal ones. This has now been exposed for the myth that it is. It's a well-proven fact that all female orgasms stem, directly or indirectly, from the clitoris. It is perhaps difficult for a man to accept that his penis may not be the source of all womanly pleasures (which is perhaps how the vaginal-orgasm-is-best myth grew up), but if a man wants to be a competent lover, he'll concentrate far more on the clitoris than the vagina.

'Should I fake orgasm?'

A lot of people do, and you don't have to be into amateur dramatics to do it. A few well-timed moans and grunts, some skilful use of the genital muscles and a little rapid panting can fool all but the most experienced lovers. And men are just as capable of feigning orgasm as women. Contrary to popular belief, a woman cannot always tell if her partner ejaculates because the inner part of her vagina is not over-supplied with nerve endings.

Why the deception? Sometimes it's done to spare a partner's feelings ('He/she will feel bad if I don't come'). Sometimes it can be a sign of deeper psycho-sexual difficulties. But if someone's been putting a lot of effort into making you come, and it's important to him or her that you do, or if you just want to get the whole thing over and done with as quickly as possible, the temptation to fake can be quite strong.

'Don't' is the short answer. You may tell yourself you're faking for your partner's sake, but what you're really doing is selling both of you short. You deny yourself the opportunity to increase your pleasure and you deny your partner the opportunity to improve the relationship. And if you fake once, you might have to keep on faking. Your partner will feel that he or she is pressing all the right buttons! How will he or she ever find out about the others?

Low self-esteem often lies at the root of the temptation to fake orgasm. Fakers prefer to keep up appearances rather than admit to themselves and their partners what gives them most pleasure. So by all means show your partner you enjoy making love, but don't pretend you've been to the moon and back if you haven't! It's fairer to both of you to be honest. If your lovemaking doesn't live up to expectations, there's something that needs ironing out, not covering up.

'Does orgasm really matter?'

Sex should be enjoyed for its own sake, and the best part is often the wanting and not the satisfaction. Orgasms should not be compulsively sought at the cost of relaxing and enjoying being intimate. A lot of the pleasure of sex comes from other things besides intercourse itself. It is comforting to be close to another warm body, rewarding to give pleasure even if you don't get it back in kind, and satisfying to know that your partner is prepared to do the same for you.

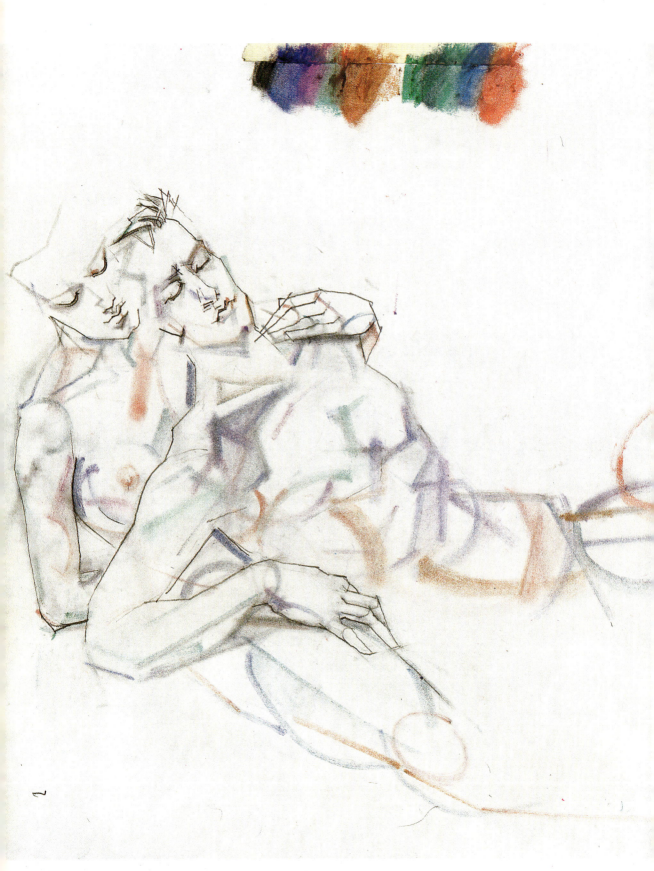

7
And so to bed...

Young people today have more options open to them than their parents or grandparents did. In the bad old days (or the good old days, depending on which way you look at it) the stoppers on sex were a fear of pregnancy, a belief that sex outside of marriage was wrong, and the idea that all women should go to the altar as virgins.

Today, more liberal attitudes towards sexuality, and easier access to contraception, have removed many of the traditional reasons for chastity. So that when and whether to have sex has become a very personal decision. Apart from the legal ban on a man or boy having sex with a girl he knows to be under 16, there are very few formal guidelines laid down as to when we should start to have sexual relationships. This puts the responsibility squarely on the shoulders of the individual, which is as it should be. But all this freedom means that we're free to have sex for the wrong reasons as well as the right ones.

The First Time

Sex is one of the milestones we all pass on the way to adulthood, but if others brag about having passed it, it may begin to feel like a millstone for those who haven't. There's a natural temptation to be like the rest, to keep up, not to miss out. Often it's only with the wisdom of hindsight that we see that conformity may not have been the best of reasons for sex.

Vicky, Paul and Caroline are now in their early twenties but this is the way they now see their first sexual experiences. (They talked openly and privately into a tape recorder without being prompted or observed.)

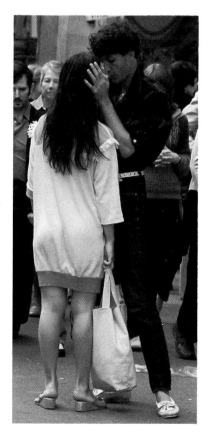

PAUL *'I was 15 but I told everyone I was 13. I thought the younger I was the better it sounded — to show off to my friends. I said "I've done it, and it was great". Actually it was terrible. It was all preplanned. I went and bought a Durex on the station. I wanted to lose my virginity because all my friends said they had. I thought at the end of it, I thought "Christ, is that it! Is that what it's all about!" I told my friends the same day. I didn't feel anything for her really. I just wanted to have sex. I didn't think of the girl, she was just for sex.'*

VICKY *'I remember when I first "did it". It was...just anyone, not someone I particularly liked. Well, I did quite fancy him, but I just wanted to do it. I remember rushing off afterwards and telling everyone.'*

And so to bed . . .

CAROLINE *'I didn't tell anyone immediately afterwards because I was in a year at school where everyone was either a year or 18 months older than me and they'd all done it. They were really into all that kind of stuff. I felt really left out, so I just did it with someone who was an old family friend I sort of quite liked. We'd grown up together and everything, and we were put in the same bedroom one Christmas holiday and we just did it. It was all very responsible. He managed to sneak downstairs to his father's washbag and get a Durex. I didn't know what it was.'*

VICKY *'Didn't you? Did you feel guilty?'*

CAROLINE *'I suppose I did in a funny way, yes. Because the first thing I did was just jump into a bath and sit in it for hours and hours! I didn't do it for another two years after the first time. It was just like...let's get it over and done with. At least it's done now.'*

VICKY *'Yes, I remember it being really fumbly. I do actually remember that it did quite hurt. I didn't want to say. I thought "I can't say anything. I've got to act as if it's OK." It took two minutes — yes, about two minutes — then it was all over. That's all it was to me. Sort of sweaty and uncomfortable.'*

CAROLINE *'I don't think he'd ever done it before. Actually, at the time, I thought "It's funny that someone who hasn't done it before knows exactly what to do." That's exactly what was going through my head. I didn't think about me at all. I just thought "This is really boring". I thought it was all meant for a man to have fun.'*

VICKY *'Exactly.'*

CAROLINE *'You just lie there.'*

PAUL *'I didn't think of the girl. I didn't think, well, is she getting an orgasm or anything. No. I just thought "Right I'm going to come". Just like that.'*

VICKY *'Yes, that's all I remember for ages. Every time you just lay there and that was it and it was over. You didn't actually do anything either really.'*

Vicky, Paul and Caroline haven't been scarred in any way by their early experiences; they've all grown up able to enjoy sex with partners they trust and care for. But all three have changed their attitudes and now admit to feeling guilty and not a little shocked by their earlier behaviour.

ROMANTIC IMAGES OF LOVE AND SEX (BELOW AND OPPOSITE) IN MAGAZINES, NEWSPAPERS, IN THE MOVIES AND ON TV HAVE GIVEN US A LOT TO LIVE UP TO.

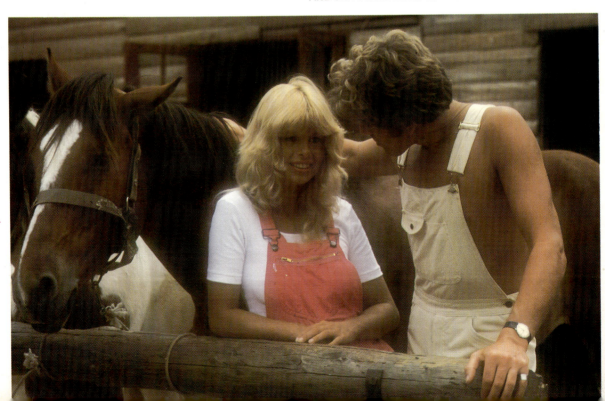

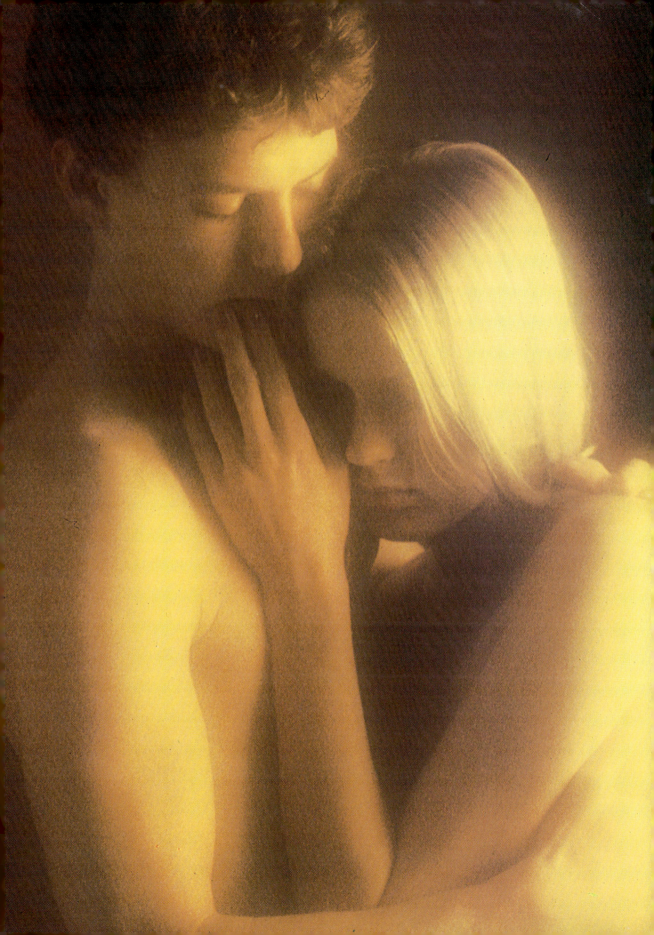

And so to bed . . .

Clearly, early sexual experiences don't always live up to expectations. If you have sex just to keep up with your friends, or simply to get it over with, or out of sheer curiosity, the outcome is likely to be disappointing, and what should have been a memorable event becomes a rather empty, fleeting experience.

So sex shouldn't be seen as a race for the start. A competitive spirit is not a good basis for satisfying sex. No one should feel pressurized into sex by others before he or she is ready, and no one should pressurize anyone else into it. The possible damage to feelings is too great.

'I'd only known him a couple of weeks. I was 16. I did it because my friend was having sex with her

schoolteacher and she kept telling me how nice it was and how I should do it and how she'd fix me up with his friend. I felt really pressured by her. Then I met this man on the beach. It sounds dreadful, but I did know him to say hello to. We went out a couple of times and then he took me to bed. We didn't discuss it beforehand, but I knew that this was going to be it.

He was in his late twenties. I didn't enjoy it at all at the time. It hurt and I bled a lot. You need to be able to trust someone. You need to know they're not going to use you and leave you, which was the fear I had, and which is exactly what happened. The first time you have sex with someone, you need to feel certain of that person, that they're still going to be there afterwards, that it's you they

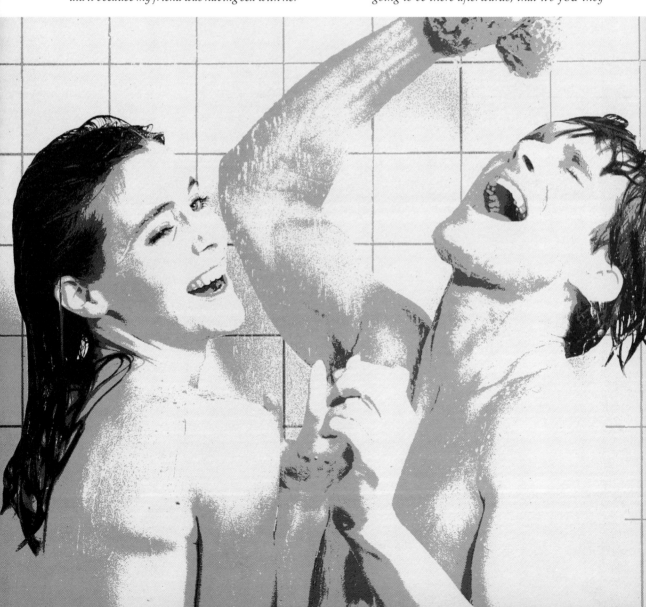

love and not just that they want to get you into bed or that you're a virgin conquest, which is very much what I felt.' JILL

There is no legal age at which we *should* start having sexual relationships. Biologically, we may be physically mature from the age of around 13 onwards. Legally it is a different matter. There is no minimum age of sexual consent for boys, though there is for girls — it's 16.

Most people agree that sex gets better with time and practice. For good sex, you need a relaxed and comfortable setting, plenty of good feelings about yourself, and a partner you can trust. The chances of having all or any of these things greatly increase as we get older. Self-esteem — placing a high value on your own worth — is a quality which is particularly likely to

develop with age, and is absolutely vital to good sexual relationships. If you don't value yourself highly enough, you'll sell yourself short in relationships, settle for less than ideal treatment from your partner, and not be firm enough about saying what you want and what pleases you. Few people in their early teens have the self-esteem to know what they want and ask for it.

In this sense, first-time-ever-sex has some parallels with sex-for-the-first-time-with-a-new-partner. You're unlikely to respond unless you're relaxed, and you're unlikely to feel relaxed with someone you don't feel close to. It isn't just a question of time, either. There are people we feel very close to almost immediately; others we never really get close to. But generally, the longer you've known someone the better able you'll feel to let down the defences.

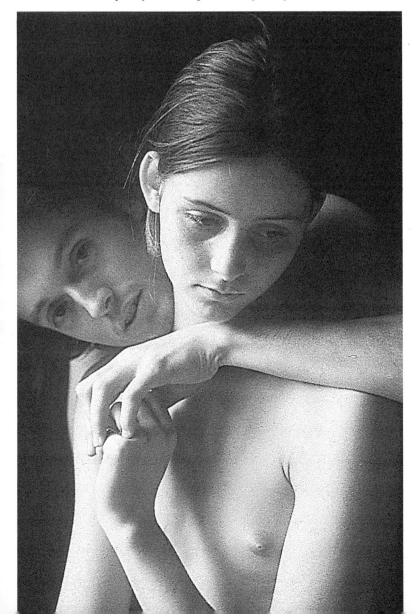

A COMBINATION OF FUN, TENDERNESS AND RESPONSIBILITY: THAT'S WHAT MAKING LOVE IS ALL ABOUT.

The one-night stand

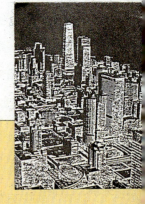

How does it happen? How is it that you can go out for an evening's drinking, dancing or party-going and end up in a comparative stranger's bed? Usually drink has a lot to do with it. Alcohol is probably the greatest ally of casual sex. It shortens the memory and silences the spoilsport voice of conscience. It also has a way of beating down reserve, removing inhibitions and inducing a state of euphoria which can be mistaken for the Real Thing. In short, a drink over the odds can transform a perfectly ordinary human being into the most captivating charmer.

If all one-night stands started off in the cold light of the morning after, they'd almost certainly never happen! Seen through hung-over eyes, last night's catch will revert back, Cinderella-like, to Mr or Ms Average. The sheer awkwardness and embarrassment which invariably set in when the alcohol wears off can blight the most promising relationship. What should be romantic drama turns into situation comedy.

It's a lot to expect a budding relationship to survive the seamier side of the morning after — sweaty bodies and less-than-sweet breath, stale aftershave and perfume. Not to mention practical anxieties about pregnancy and the possibility of infection. Unless you know a person very well indeed, there is no tactful way of asking whether he or she has a clean bill of health (see Chapter 12). And there's a double dilemma concerning contraception: if you carry your method with you, it looks as if you preplanned the whole thing: forget it, and you risk the consequences.

A lot of one-night stands happen because people are lonely; they want intimacy and affection, but all they get is sex. The sad fact is that it is perfectly possible to be close to someone physically, yet be light years away emotionally. For this reason, casual sex is often thought to work against women, if only because they usually allow themselves to be more emotionally involved than men. In fact women are not always the victims nor men the victors. The man who goes in for deliberate one-night stands — there's another notch on the bedpost! — is often reassuring himself of his sexuality, and may not be able to cope with the emotional demands of a deeper relationship.

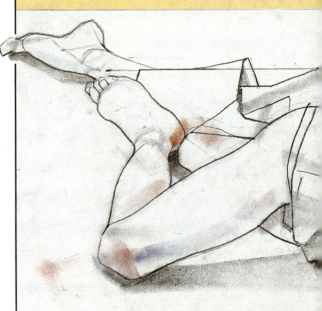

'She looks so *nice* lying there. Shouldn't really have asked her back the first time. She's here though. No brute force. Wonder if she does this sort of thing often? Doesn't look the type. Must have been the drink. She was amazing. Hope she thought the same about me . . . Wonder what she *did* think? Did I do OK? What will she think when she wakes up? Wish the room wasn't such a tip. All Pete's filthy cigarette ends lying around the place. At least the sheets are clean. Maybe she'd like a coffee, breakfast in bed even. Make a fuss of her, then we can have a bit of a chat, get things more on the level . . ."

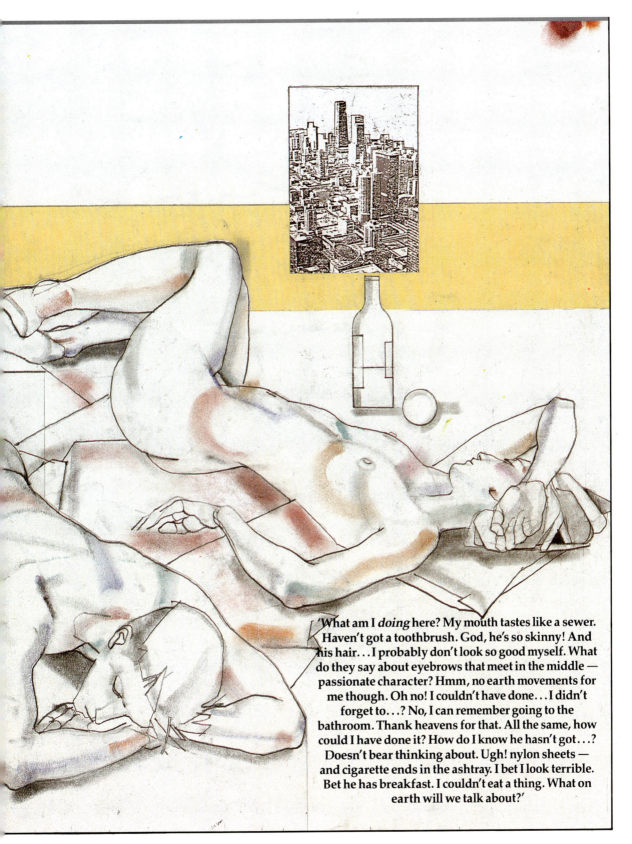

'What am I *doing* here? My mouth tastes like a sewer. Haven't got a toothbrush. God, he's so skinny! And his hair. . . I probably don't look so good myself. What do they say about eyebrows that meet in the middle — passionate character? Hmm, no earth movements for me though. Oh no! I couldn't have done. . . I didn't forget to. . .? No, I can remember going to the bathroom. Thank heavens for that. All the same, how could I have done it? How do I know he hasn't got. . .? Doesn't bear thinking about. Ugh! nylon sheets — and cigarette ends in the ashtray. I bet I look terrible. Bet he has breakfast. I couldn't eat a thing. What on earth will we talk about?'

One-off encounters are rarely satisfying sexually. After the tingling excitement of expectation, the actual experience can be a bit of a let down. Neither partner knows much about the other — what his or her likes and dislikes are. And both may have worries about 'performing' well. Good sexual relationships depend on feelings of security and trust, and these are not built up overnight.

How do you know whether a one-night stand is just that or a prelude to something more lasting? You don't. But you'll have a better idea if you've put in a little research beforehand. After all, when the first flush of passion is over, you're going to be spending more time talking and laughing together than erotically entwined in the bedroom. Erotic curiosity is fine, but try not to let it get the better of you.

Postponing sex until you've established some common ground and mutual trust means that you're less likely to be left feeling like a human cast-off. Perhaps the best deterrent to a repeat one-night stand is the empty, dejected feeling after the first one. But that's learning the hard way.

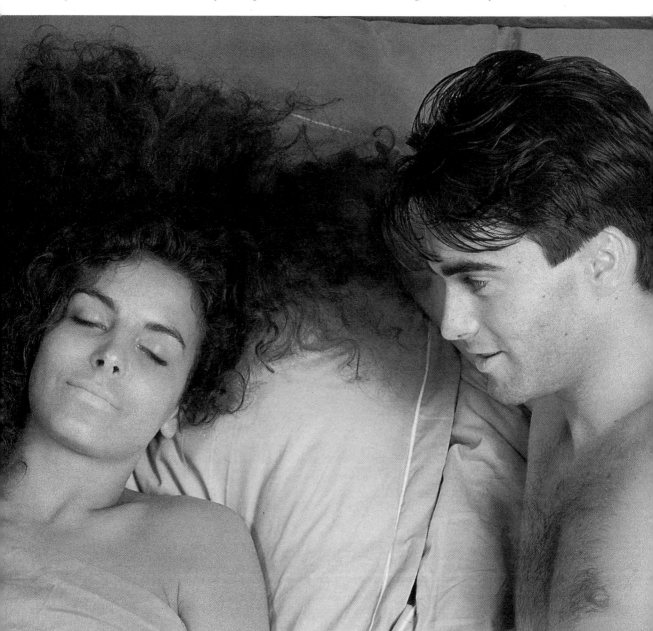

And so to bed . . .

WILL YOUR ONE-NIGHT STAND LEAD TO A MORE
PERMANENT RELATIONSHIP? LACK OF FEELINGS OF
SECURITY AND TRUST OFTEN RESULT IN EARLY
BREAK-UPS.

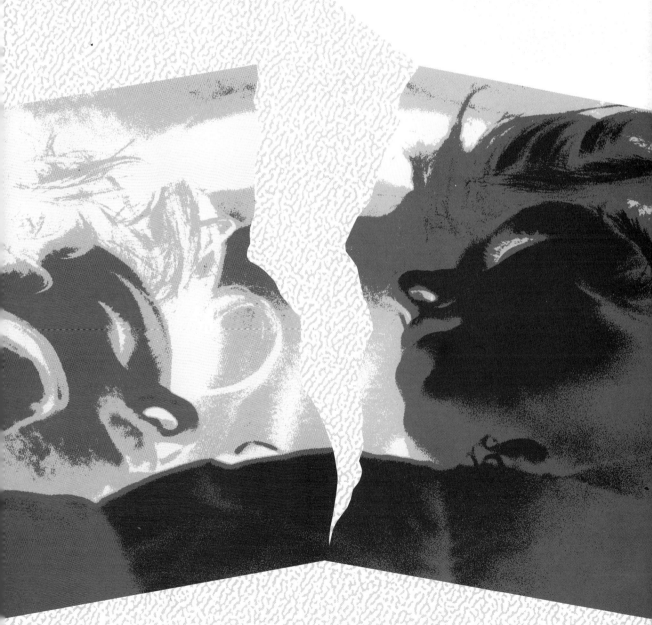

Great expectations _____

We expect a lot more from our sexual experiences today than our grandparents did. Gone are the days when women were taught to lie back and think of green fields and men had to put up with log-like partners. It's now accepted that women have sexual appetites every bit as large as those of men, and every right to have them satisfied. So it's not surprising that men feel the pressure on them to perform. Sex manuals to improve technique and performance are outsold only by cookery books; agony columns are full of letters from people asking how to be better lovers.

Too much emphasis on performance, however, can have a bad effect on our sex lives. What should be an area of relaxation and closeness between men and women becomes yet another arena in which we feel the need to prove ourselves. Sex begins to feel more like work than pleasure. 'We had sex three times' or 'She had three orgasms' gets to sound like 'I got three A grades' or 'I scored three goals'.

Part of the problem may be that the goals we set ourselves are unrealistic. 'Bodice-ripping' fiction has a lot to answer for in this respect. Take this torrid episode from Harold Robbins' novel *The Betsy*.

'She began to climax almost before he was fully inside her. Then she couldn't stop them, one coming rapidly after the other as he slammed into her with the force of the giant body press she had seen working in his factory. . . And finally, when orgasm after orgasm had racked her body into a searing sheet of flame and she could bear it no more, she cried out to him . . . A roar came from deep inside his throat and his hands tightened on her breasts. She half screamed and her hands grabbed into the hair of his chest. Then all his weight seemed to fall in on her, crushing the breath from her body, and as she felt the hot onrushing gushes of his semen turning her insides into viscous flowing lava she discovered herself climaxing again.'

YOUNG PEOPLE ARE OFTEN CONFUSED ABOUT WHAT TO EXPECT FROM RELATIONSHIPS . . . GLOSSY CELLULOID IMAGES (RIGHT) ARE OFTEN TO BLAME.

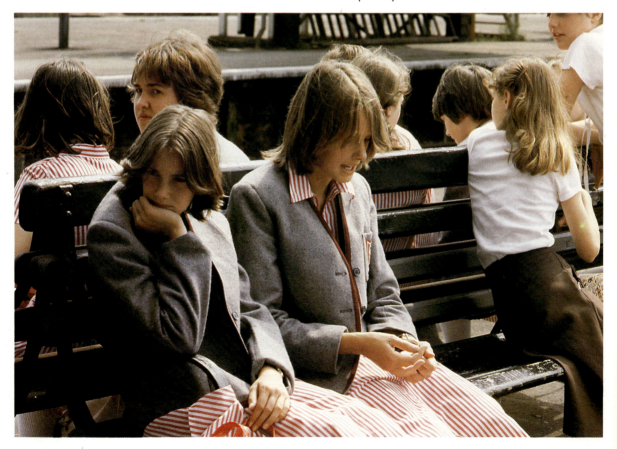

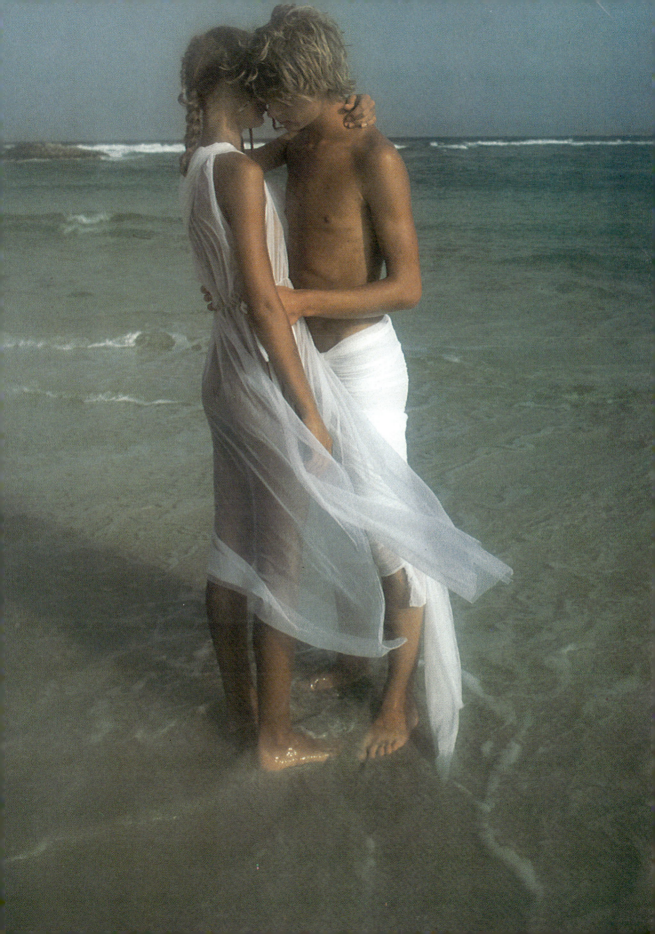

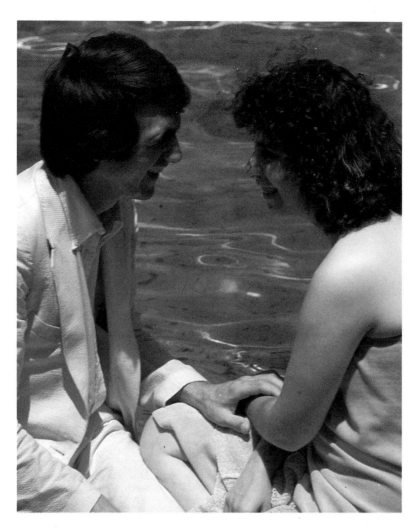

SOME SEX GUIDES SUGGEST THERE IS A FOOL-PROOF AROUSAL FORMULA FOR EVERYONE. BUT BLUEPRINT SEX USUALLY MEANS BORING SEX. WHAT WORKS FOR ONE PERSON DOESN'T NECESSARILY WORK FOR ANOTHER.

Few of us can expect to reach these peaks of passion. Yet these are often the standards we use to measure our equipment, our performance and our satisfaction levels. Men feel they're expected to produce orgasms (preferably multiple) to order in their partner, and women feel they've let their man down if they can't oblige. Unfortunately, these anxieties can be self-fulfilling. Worrying about impotence and about not reaching a climax can actually cause these problems. Listen to the anxiety in this account from Helen, an 18-year-old college student.

'It was a shame really, we started off all right. I really fancied him and had done for ages, so I was quite excited. He turned out to be very experienced in a sort of way that was a bit of a turn off. I kept thinking "Who did he learn all this with? Does he expect what worked with the last girl to work with me?" I'd have preferred us to learn together, I suppose. Anyway, he certainly made me feel inferior, a bit green. I tried to enjoy what

was going on but my mind kept floating off thinking about how badly I was doing. It was as if my mind was standing over my body saying "Go on, he's trying hard enough to make you respond, you could at least show you're grateful". But the more he seemed to be watching my reactions the more I concentrated on them and the quicker they disappeared. When I felt the pressure was on, my body switched off. The harder I tried to make myself come, the worse it got. At one point, he broke off and asked what was wrong with me. But I couldn't bring myself to tell him what I wanted him to do. Earlier, I'd moved his hand just a fraction because he was hurting me and he tensed up straight away.

After that things really went downhill. I wouldn't have minded myself. Probably it would have come right in the end if we'd stopped thinking about it. As it turned out, I didn't get another chance. He obviously couldn't cope with us not being a success and said there wasn't much point in us seeing each other if we weren't compatible.'

'Left hand down and a little to the right'____

Perhaps because of all this emphasis on performance, we seem to have become obsessed with finding ways of improving our sexual technique. A great deal of time and effort in recent years has been put into tracking down and identifying our super-sensitive body zones. In books with titles like *The Sex Atlas, The Techniques of Sex* and *How to be a Better Lover,* the sexual mapmakers have plotted these for us, together with detailed instructions on how to find and titillate them. The message is that all of us can have bigger and better orgasms, make them last longer, and generally scale Robbins-style heights just by pressing the right buttons.

Technique has its place in lovemaking, but it's not everything. We are not machines programmed to twitch and pant and pulsate at the touch of buttons, but complex beings with our own individual whims and wants, fads and fancies. The intrinsic problems with 'how-to-do-it' guides is that they suggest there is a fool-proof arousal formula which can be used on virtually everyone. They ignore the fact that there are no two people alike — what works for one person doesn't necessarily work for another. Some people like to have their ears fondled, others their toes. Some like slow, gentle lovemaking; others get excited by a faster more forceful approach.

Besides, why read up in theory what you can find out in practice? Blueprint sex is boring sex. A one-sided stress on the physical side turns what should be an exciting process of mutual discovery, into a routine, albeit pleasant, mechanical exercise. Reading too many books on sex techniques is a bit like reading too many books on car maintenance: you don't want to get so bogged down with what might go wrong that you don't enjoy the drive.

No matter how experienced we are, nor how many books we've read, we have to learn from each other. There's no way of knowing beforehand what will please your partner, no reason why you should feel you should know, and no nicer way of finding out than through trial and error. A good lover is not one who knows what to do, but who knows how to ask.

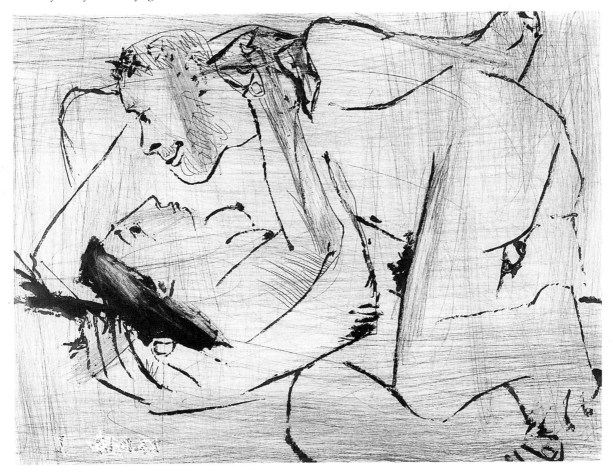

Talking about sex

The best way of finding out what pleases someone is to ask. If you feel paralysed by the thought of asking your partner what to do, you're not alone. Lots of people find it difficult to ask, and just as difficult to tell. They feel they ought to know intuitively what to do, that being told is a criticism of what they have been doing.

The problem seems to be worse for men than women. Men may talk a lot about sex — risqué jokes, allusions to sexual prowess — but underneath the bravado, how much real communication is going on? A Real Man (here he is again) is supposed to know what women want and be able to provide it. Some women keep this myth alive by clinging to the belief that if they have to tell their lovers what pleases them, sex will lose its spontaneity.

This is obviously quite silly. We're none of us mind readers and we're all of us different. Everyone has their own needs and moods, sensitive spots and no-go areas. To enjoy sex together you have to share this information with your partner, and encourage him or her to do the same. What's the point of going through a relationship stuck in patterns of mutually unsatisfying sexual habits, not daring to tell each other what your

needs really are? If you stay stuck too long, the chances are high that one or both of you will lose interest sexually, and that you'll start to look for another sexual partner.

Of course, declaring any kind of want is an uncomfortably self-revealing act for some people. But saying what you want is important in every area of life — it's not selfish or unreasonable. And in the area of sex, stored up resentments stemming from unmet or unexpressed wants are a sure-fire way of crippling a relationship.

It's odd that an activity as natural as sex isn't discussed more frankly and openly — at least not in Western society. Imagine what it would be like if it were considered indelicate to talk about eating, so that two people didn't dare to tell each other they were hungry for fear of giving offence. Or that every night they sat down to liver and bacon when what they really preferred was omelette and chips one night and ravioli another, but they couldn't bring themselves to talk about it! For food read sex, and you begin to get some idea of the folly of not communicating sexual likes and dislikes.

BODY LANGUAGE CAN BE EFFECTIVELY USED TO COMMUNICATE SEXUAL PREFERENCES.

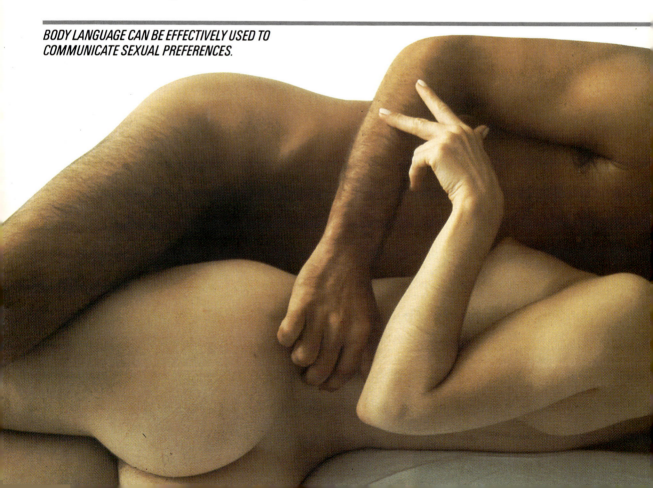

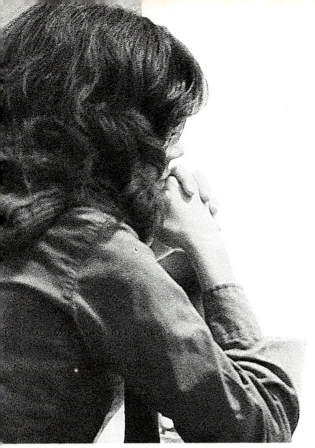

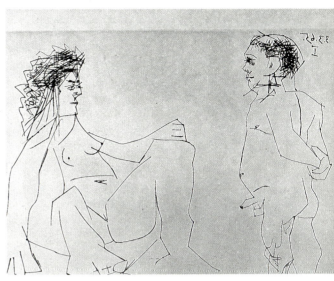

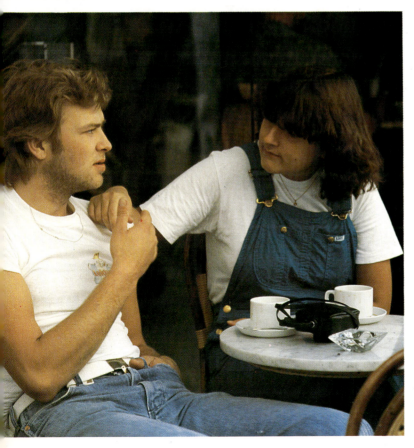

TALKING ABOUT SEX IS A POPULAR PASTIME FOR MANY PEOPLE. BUT BETWEEN PARTNERS ANY REAL COMMUNICATION OF WANTS IS OFTEN SADLY LACKING. A GOOD LOVER KNOWS HOW TO ASK.

Why should sex be so difficult to talk about? Partly it's because we don't have the right words. Words are always a poor substitute for deep and powerful feelings, but the words we have just aren't satisfactory. Our sexual vocabulary is better suited to the bar room, the doctor's surgery or a village tea party than the bedroom. Slang terms — like 'cunt', 'fuck', 'prick' and so on — may seem too degrading and coarse; medical terms — like 'vagina', 'intercourse' and 'penis' — too cold and clinical; and euphemisms — like 'private parts' and 'sleeping together' — too coy and inexact.

Another difficulty for some people is that talking about sex leads to a degree of intimacy or self-disclosure that they find disturbing; they're afraid to take the lid off their fantasies or let the depth of their feelings show. But another person's fantasies (more on these on page 128) and feelings can be a turn on!

So how do you go about expressing your wants and feelings? Remember you're not expressing them in the spirit of complaint or criticism. You're doing it because you care about the relationship. The watchword is candour, but candour with sensitivity. Here are some basic guidelines.

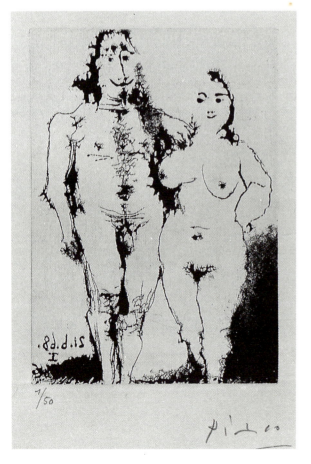

■ **Know what it is you want.** Unless you can communicate your sexual needs to yourself, you'll find it difficult to pass them on to someone else. This means being familiar with your own body, your specially sensitive zones, your preferred tempo. Read the section on masturbation on page 124.

■ **Pick the right moment.** At the time you're actually making love, the atmosphere might be too emotionally charged for constructive discussion. Talking beforehand or waiting till afterwards can take the steam out of the situation. Talking about sex before you get started can be a nice warm-up! And doing so afterwards needn't take the form of a post mortem; talking about things you've just done can be a turn on in its own right.

■ **Aim for positive reinforcement.** In other words, pick up on the plus points. Don't say *'You never...'* (You never undress me/let me take the lead/want to do anything different). Substitute *'I'd love you to...'* for *'You never...'* and notice the difference. Praise works better than criticism. For every time you say 'Shall we try...' or 'I'd like it if...', make sure there are three times when you say something like 'wasn't it nice when...' or 'I love it when you...'

■ **Avoid long words and cool logic.** Develop your own intimate and private terms for lovemaking and don't be afraid to be a little direct and earthy. When they're sexually aroused many people like to use (and hear) words and phrases they might not use in their everyday language. Words which sound vulgar in another context can be transformed in sex, so you should feel neither offended nor inhibited. Taboo words can spring some erotic surprises!

■ **Use body language.** Communication needn't always be verbal. There are many ways of relaying sexual messages through gestures and movements: a hand on your lover's shoulder, for example, to say 'speed up' or 'slow down'; taking his or her hand and guiding it to a more sensitive area of your body, and making noises which say 'that feels good'; tracing a pattern with your fingertips on your partner's body which he or she then uses as a guide to placing and pacing his or her caresses.

TALKING ABOUT SEX BEFORE YOU GET STARTED CAN BE A NICE WARM-UP.

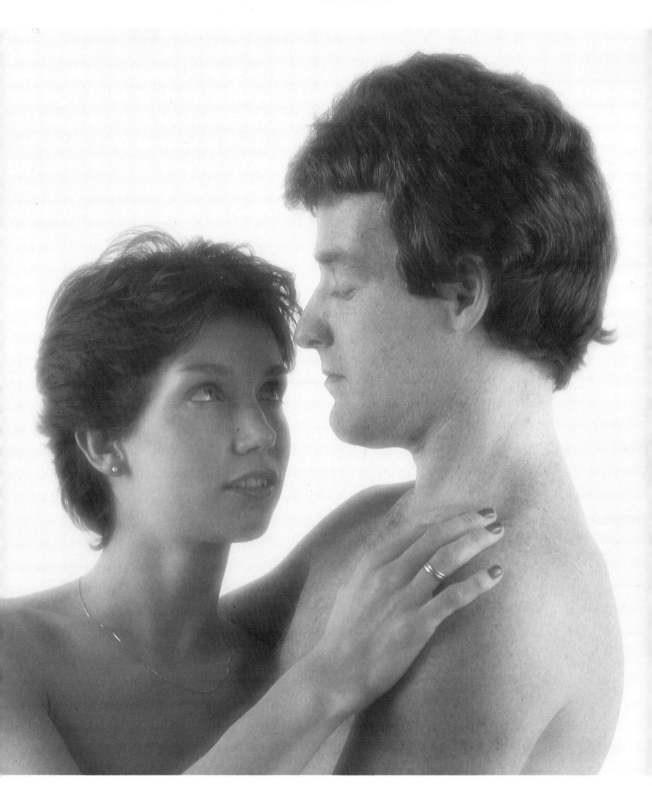

And so to bed . . .

Your mind is your biggest sex organ

A sex therapist once said that sex was composed of friction and fantasy. Good sex is about physical and mental feelings and both mind and body need stimulating if we're to respond. Though it's our bodily sensations we're most conscious of in sex, it's important to remember that it's the mind that is the prime mover. If your head is blocking those sensations, the best technique in the world will not arouse you. Sexual excitement and sensual enjoyment tend to short-circuit whenever unpleasant feelings are around — guilt, anger or anxiety, for example — and bottling up those feelings can make things worse (see page 167). One of the answers is talking, about the feelings themselves, about the wants that are not being met.

The irony is that most of the mental states that are essential to satisfying sex are precisely those that are discouraged in other areas of behaviour. When you're making love you have to let yourself go, take down the fences, lose your grip, make yourself vulnerable, and do whatever comes naturally. All this wild abandon goes very much against the grain, against what we have been taught. In sex, we have to unlearn most of the responses that normally make us feel comfortable. And until we gain sexual experience we feel insecure. And when we feel insecure it is very natural to ask 'Am I normal?' So read on.

YOUR BODY SENSATIONS TEND TO SHORT CIRCUIT IN THE PRESENCE OF DESTRUCTIVE FEELINGS LIKE GUILT OR ANGER. TRY TO MAKE YOUR MIND WORK FOR YOUR BODY INSTEAD OF AGAINST IT.

And so to bed . . .

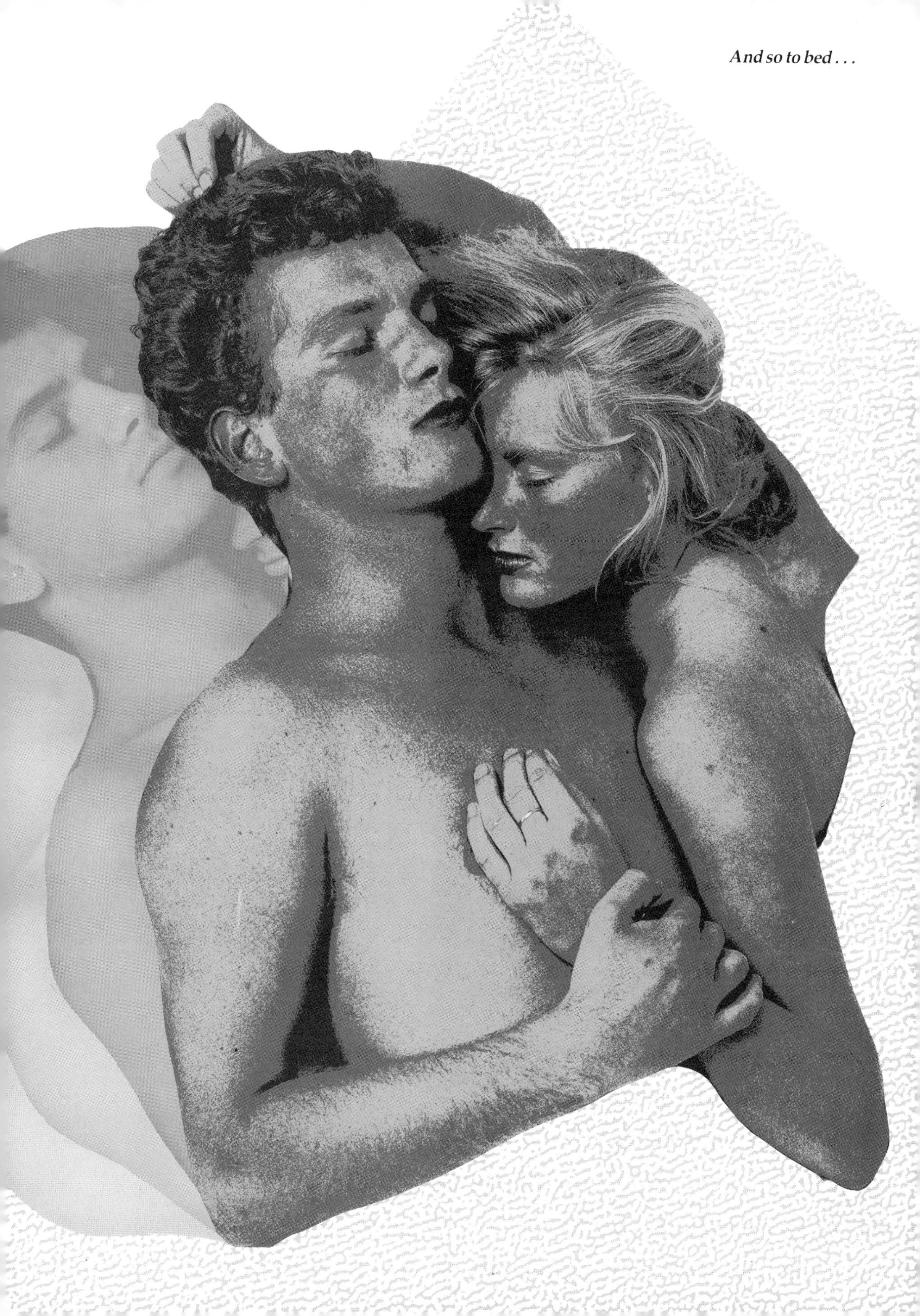

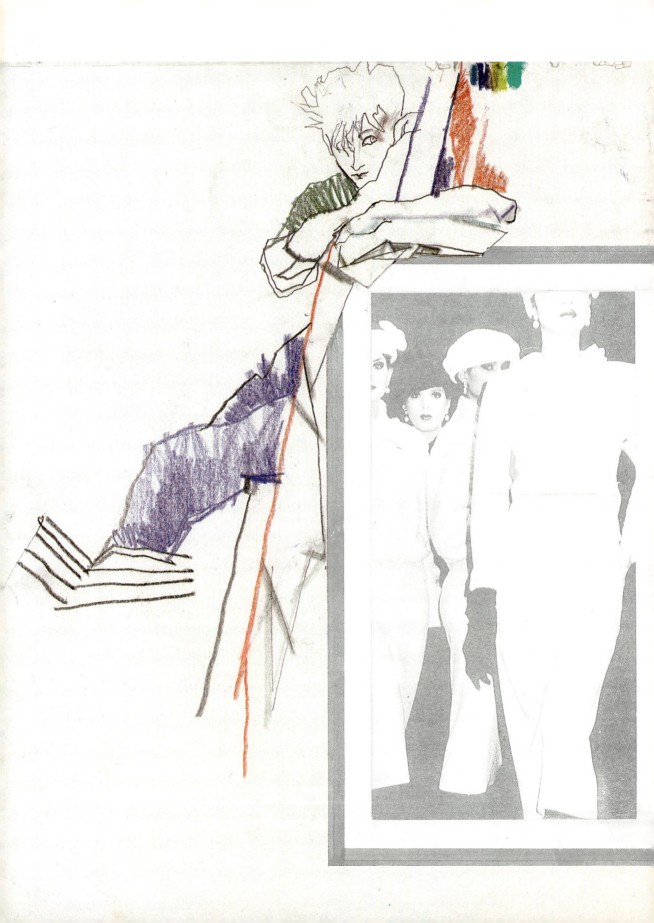

8

Am I normal?

Is the size of my penis normal? The fact that I like oral sex? That I masturbate? That I have sex twice a night/once a month/upside down/on the back of a motorbike? You name it, people will worry about it if they think they're out of line — at least, as far as sex is concerned they will. We strive to be different and unique in other areas of behaviour, but in sexual matters we seem to be obsessed with being normal!

But what is normal? Is it simply a question of being average? In the statistical sense of the word, normal is the way the majority of people around us act, or appear to. So, if ninety-nine people do something and one doesn't, is that person abnormal?

Beware statistics!_____

The problem is, of course, particularly in the realms of sexual behaviour, that no one is at all sure exactly what it is that other people do. Our sexual habits are rarely spoken about, even less often seen, and they're often the subject of untruths and cover-ups. Sex surveys may tell us that masturbation is common practice, that most people have sexual fantasies, and that the average man thinks about sex at least six times a day, but you won't get people admitting these things to each other. The result is that most of us, on occasion, imagine we're the only person in the world doing something that is in fact extremely common.

Statistics may, occasionally, be reassuring but they can also be harmful. The numbers say that it's normal to be heterosexual because something like nine out of ten people prefer partners of the opposite sex. But we can't say the one in ten who doesn't is not normal. Only 5 per cent of people cycle to work — one in twenty — but that doesn't make all cyclists abnormal, any more than opera lovers, animal rights campaigners, or members of any other minority group are abnormal.

Are there right and proper ways to behave? The kinds of behaviour which become most common tend to be those that are morally approved of. And what gets approved of morally tends to be what fits in best in our society. If we want to raise stable, well-adjusted children, it's best not to swap or collect partners like postage stamps. One of the tenets of Christianity is that sex is for producing babies. This has traditionally ruled out practices like masturbation, oral sex, anal sex and homosexual sex because they cannot lead to pregnancy.

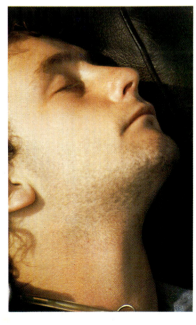

But it's backwards-way-round logic to claim that because sex is necessary to keep the human race going, the sole purpose of sex is reproduction. You might just as well say that since food is necessary to keep the body going, the sole purpose of eating is to stay alive! — which won't convince anyone who enjoys strawberry cheesecake. If the only purpose of sex were reproduction, Nature would have arranged for human females to come on heat only twice a year — ample opportunity to reproduce the species.

Also, what is statistically normal doesn't always line up with what is morally normal or sanctioned by law. One study of the sex lives of American men and women found that the practices of more than half the people questioned were actually illegal. Social attitudes and the laws that enshrine them change of course when enough people find the current rules too much of a straitjacket. Sex before marriage is a case in point; so is masturbation and homosexuality. Until people were prepared to admit to these practices, they were thought of as deviant. If social rules and taboos are so powerful that people can't feel free to bring their sexual preferences out in the open, they stay in the closet, where they do far more harm than good.

Personal preferences_____

Fortunately, masturbation and oral sex are no longer considered sinful or sick, homosexuals are no longer classified as perverts, and those who indulge in sex outside of marriage are no longer regarded as deviant.

The fact is that how you enjoy sex is purely a matter of personal preference, and is no one else's business but your own and your partner's. It is not a matter of dividing things up into right or wrong, common or uncommon, but of deciding what works best for you, always providing that neither you nor your partner is being harmed, insulted or offended.

'If I felt very uncomfortable doing something then I wouldn't do it. I wouldn't say it was abnormal, just because I didn't want to do it. If someone wanted to tie me up and put me on a bed of nails with an onion in my mouth, I'd think it was weird, obviously, but if I like doing something and my partner doesn't think I'm odd, there's no reason why I shouldn't.' JANE

'It's different for different people. It might be wrong for me but quite OK for someone else. Partly, it's the way you're brought up. It depends on your background and the type of people you've mixed with. Where I come from — South Africa — we have pretty narrow views. No girlie magazines or pin-ups. Absolutely nothing. It's surprising to come here and find everything so open. I just personally feel, it's what's right for you. It's not whether other people do it. This way or that way, it's whether you're happy with it.' MIKE

Just as no two people have exactly the same taste in food or clothes, so no two people like exactly the same things in bed. If you think you are outside the range of common activities, you shouldn't think of yourself as abnormal. Human beings are born with myriad possibilities for satisfying their sexual urges, and the possibilities you explore are normal for *you*. That said, we tend to be far more tolerant of our own whims and fancies than of others. Perversions is the name we give to *other* people's variations; our own we call preferences.

HOW YOU ENJOY SEX — EITHER WITH A PARTNER OR BY YOURSELF — IS A MATTER OF PERSONAL PREFERENCE AND IS NO ONE ELSE'S BUSINESS BUT YOUR OWN.

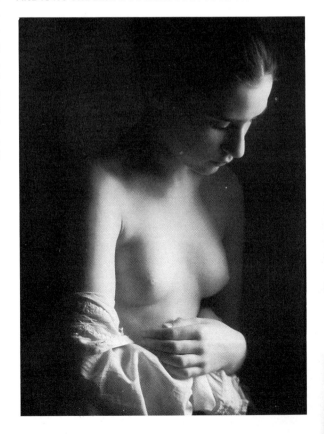

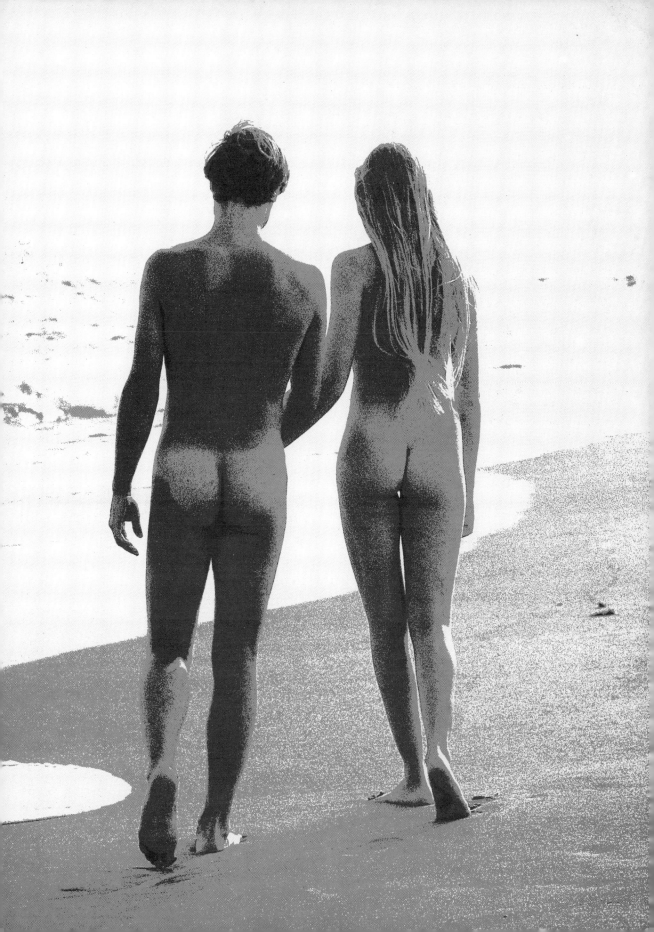

Is my sexual equipment normal?

Men and women feel inadequate about all sorts of bits of their anatomy. Here we're going to concentrate on just two items of sexual equipment, penises and breasts, because they're the subject of more hang-ups than any other.

One of the cherished illusions men have about their sexual performance is that the bigger their penis the better they'll satisfy their partners. It's an illusion that has been nourished by pulp fiction. The kind of men you read about in Harold Robbins or Judith Krantz novels have penises as hard as iron and as long as barbers' poles, indomitably poised for action. As soon as they lose one erection, there's another at the ready. Rarely do you come across floppy or diminutive penises, the kind that wilt a little and need coaxing into action.

As a result, men in real life (as opposed to Real Men) examine their own equipment and wonder whether it measures up. One of the problems is that you always see your own penis from above (unless you look in a mirror), from which perspective it looks foreshortened. In fact, despite all the fears (and boasts) to the contrary, penis size does not vary markedly from one man to the next. There *are* some large penises around, just as there are some men whose erections can last a long time and return after a short time. But there is far less difference than is generally supposed. Believe it or not, some researchers have gone around with a tape measure! Penises vary in length between 2 in (5 cm) and 4 in (10 cm) when limp, but when they're erect they all average out at about 6 in (15 cm). Those that are smaller when relaxed increase in size more than larger ones. In other words, with erection, the differences tend to level out. One erect penis is much the same size as another. Besides, it is now firmly established beyond a shadow of a doubt that penis size makes not an atom of difference to women's sexual enjoyment. The vagina can stretch sideways and lengthways to accommodate any size of penis. In fact, some women complain that a really hard, long penis actually hurts a little.

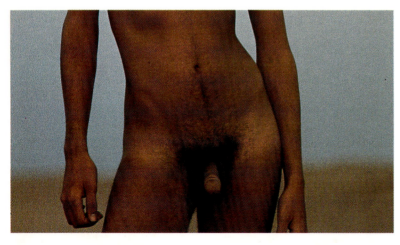

PENIS SIZE MAKES NO DIFFERENCE TO WOMEN'S SEXUAL ENJOYMENT.

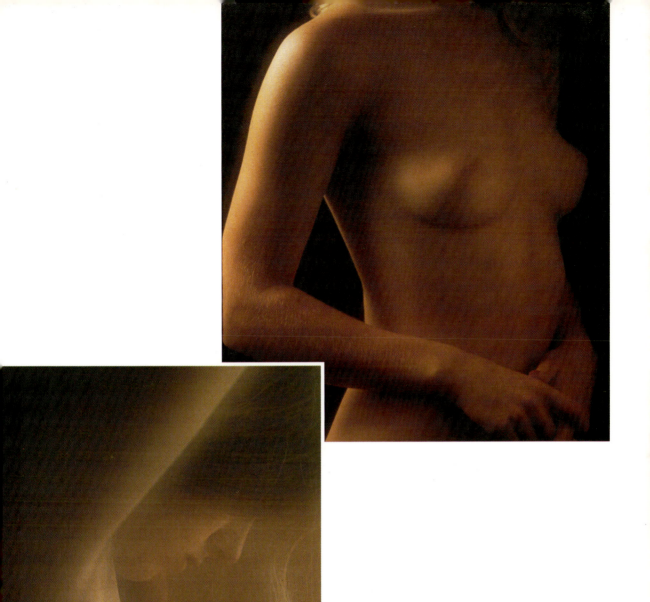

WOMEN IN MAGAZINES, ADVERTISEMENTS AND PIN-UPS HAVE PERFECTLY SHAPED BREASTS. THESE MAY BE THE IDEAL, BUT THEY'RE CERTAINLY NOT THE AVERAGE.

121

And now to breasts. There's an old saying that men are aroused through their eyes and women through their ears. Even non-sexist men, who do their best to use their ears as well, are quickly turned on by the sight of a shapely bosom. This has been a godsend for the advertising industry, but the bugbear of women. Women in glossy magazines, advertisements and pin-ups have perfectly shaped breasts, and neat bottoms and long slim legs too. These may be the ideals, but they're certainly not average.

'I've got small breasts — you've got to look hard to see anything — and it really used to bug me. You look at these men's magazines and you never see the kind of normal-sized ones you see in changing rooms. But that's what men like — these massive boobs.

I had a real complex at 18. I went to my doctor and asked if there was any chance of me growing a bit more but he told me I'd got to accept

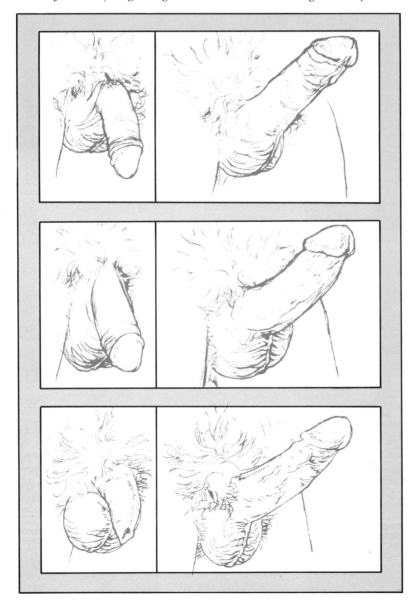

PENISES COME IN VARIOUS SHAPES AND SIZES (LEFT). NOT ALL PENISES BECOME ERECT IN THE SAME WAY, BUT WHEN THEY'RE ERECT THEY EVEN OUT TO ROUGHLY THE SAME SIZE (RIGHT).

what I'd got. Before I started to go out with Neil I'd never have dreamt of talking about it to a man. Now I couldn't give two hoots. I'm never going to be ideal but if he doesn't mind, why should I? Besides, I look at my sister. . . she's got enormous breasts and I've stood and watched men really zero in on them. Their eyes bulge towards them ignoring her face or the rest of her.' JOANNE

The point is that the busty beauties on billboards, on the big screen and in magazines are not *available*. They're there only to look at. They may be titillating images, but that's all they are. They're not flesh and blood. There's a big difference between the way you appraise someone you care for and the way you respond to a poster.

Besides, Nature is not completely cruel. Women who have bee stings for breasts are as like as not blessed with compensating factors — glossy hair, a fetching bottom, a dazzling smile.

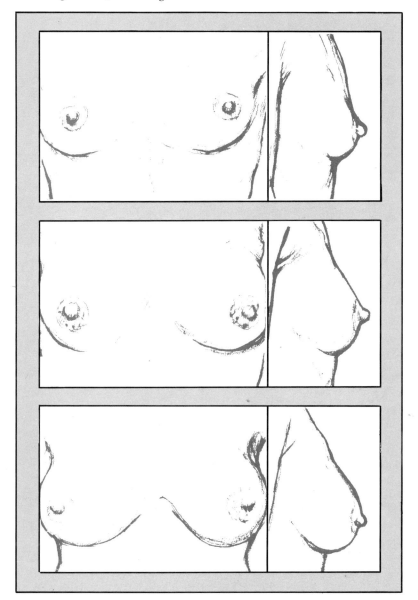

BREASTS GET FULLER AND ROUNDER THROUGH NORMAL DEVELOPMENT, BUT NOT EVERYONE ENDS UP BEING ENDOWED WITH A GENEROUS BOSOM.

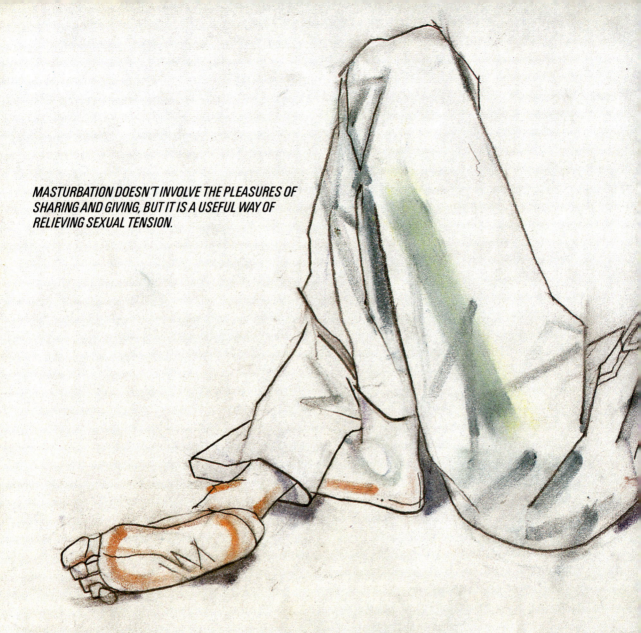

MASTURBATION DOESN'T INVOLVE THE PLEASURES OF SHARING AND GIVING, BUT IT IS A USEFUL WAY OF RELIEVING SEXUAL TENSION.

Pleasing yourself

Masturbation, the practice of finding sexual pleasure in your own body without a partner, is also known by a variety of other names which reflect the way people have tended to feel about solo sex. At the slang level, words like 'wanking', 'jerking off' and 'tossing off' describe the action in men more than women, suggesting that masturbating is not a very feminine thing to do. Other terms, like 'self-abuse', hark back to the time — comparatively recently — when masturbation was thought of as wicked and harmful. Many of the myths about masturbation that scared people witless for generations have now gone out of the window, thank goodness. Playing with yourself was supposed to make your sex organs wither and drop off, make hair grow on your palms, stunt your growth, send you mad or blind. We can laugh at these awful warnings now, but there are still books being printed which claim that anyone who masturbates regularly will find it difficult to enjoy sex with a partner.

Nothing could be further from the truth. Studies of sexual behaviour have shown that people who masturbate are more likely to have more active and satisfying sex lives than those who don't. Perhaps they're just more passionate anyway, but there's certainly no evidence that masturbation has any adverse effects on two-person sex. If there were, a lot of people's sexual relationships would be up the creek! Surveys have shown that more that 90 per cent of men and 65 per cent of women masturbate — and these percentages would be higher if everyone admitted it.

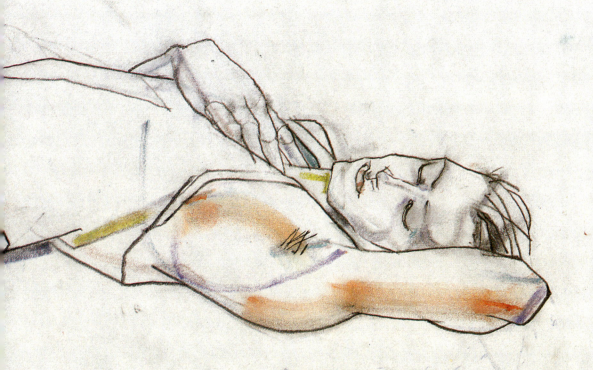

No one is better qualified than yourself to find out how your body responds. It's your head the nerve endings are connected to, so only you can know exactly what sort of stimulation your body needs in order to respond most pleasurably — how much pressure, how much tension, fast or slow…When you stimulate yourself you don't have to consider a partner's needs and responses. But when you're with a partner, you can use these insights to guide him or her to touch and stroke your body in the right place.

Some people find it deeply threatening to know that their partner masturbates. They'd prefer to think of their partner being unfaithful! But if two people feel secure enough to watch each other masturbate, they will quickly learn each other's sexual secrets.

Masturbating when you're making love (see page 134) can also get you over the hurdle of orgasm. So if it enhances enjoyment, if it doesn't offend your partner or if your partner doesn't object, you should feel free to follow your own inclinations.

Masturbation shouldn't be thought of as second best. The experience is a different one from sex with a partner. It doesn't involve the pleasures of sharing and giving, but it can be a useful way of relieving sexual tension. Many women say the orgasms they get through masturbation are often more intense than those they experience during sex with a partner. A few can only reach orgasm in this way. Pleasing yourself is not a substitute for when the real thing is not available; it's part of a wide range of sexual expression.

Rediscovering touch

Babies and small children explore and fondle their bodies quite naturally and with no shame at all, and would probably continue to do so if it were not for the fact that, as they grow up, they receive strong messages from parents and others that it is not acceptable behaviour. They may get their hands smacked, receive a scolding, or simply absorb an all-round sense of embarrassment. As they develop a sense of propriety, masturbation becomes a secret activity and sometimes stops altogether. Self-pleasuring techniques may need relearning, even if we feel shocked and self-conscious about starting up again.

Most important, the conditions must be right. You need to be relaxed, comfortable and alone, with no fear of interruption. Move your hands gently and softly over your whole body. Let your mind play on fantasies which excite you. Gradually, you can allow yourself to home in on those areas of your body where the sensations are most intense and most pleasurable.

Some men masturbate by stroking and fondling the shaft and head of the penis, or by squeezing gently and then more forcefully as excitement mounts; others lie face down and rub their bodies up and down on the bed. For most women, the usual focus of masturbation is the clitoris. Some prefer to apply direct pressure, by stroking or tweaking their clitoris with their fingers, whilst others apply more indirect pressure by rubbing the whole of the genital area, massaging rhythmically, and then faster and harder as excitement rises. Some women like to insert a finger or some other penis-shaped object into their vagina at the same time which, provided it is clean and has no sharp edges, can add to their pleasure.

Some people find that they can reach orgasm amazingly quickly by masturbating — in a matter of seconds. For others, it takes longer and it may be quite difficult to let go completely. The very experience of orgasm can be startling and disturbing if it's unexpected and unfamiliar. But it shouldn't be seen as a goal to be scored. Whether you're alone or with a partner, it's a bonus to already pleasant feelings.

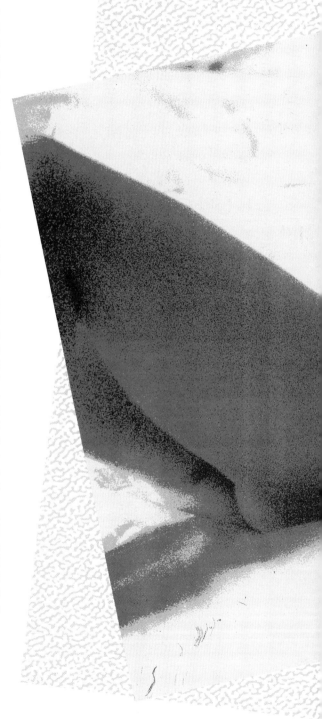

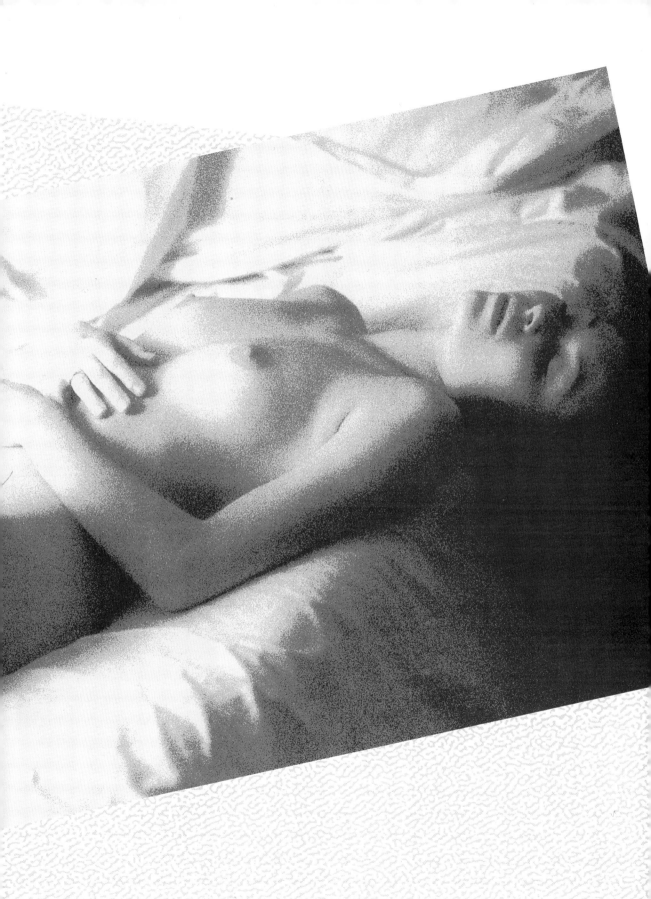

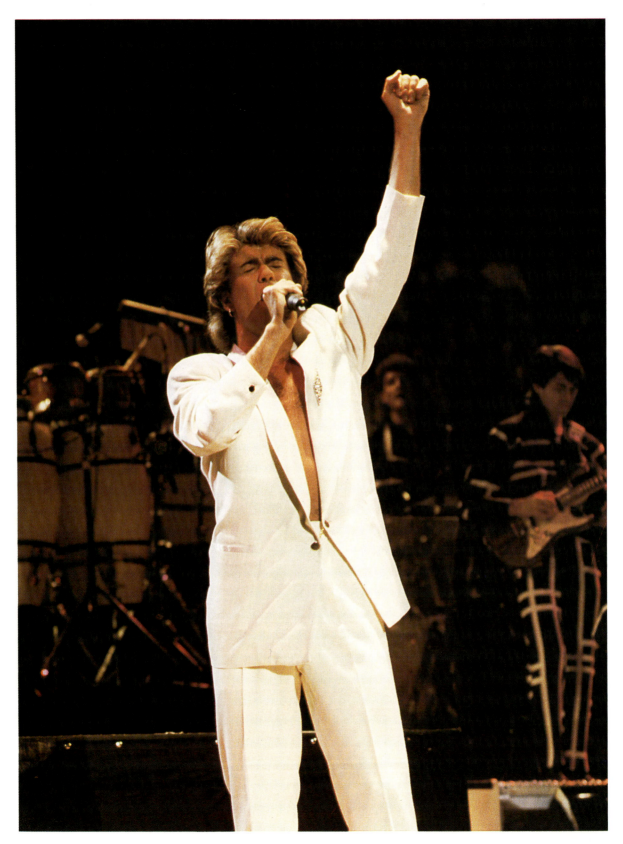

Fantasies

Everyone has fantasies. During masturbation they provide mental images to take the place of actual partners. Masturbation without fantasy would be a lonely physical exercise. But there's good evidence that most people also have erotic fantasies during lovemaking with a partner. One study of college students showed that six out of ten fantasized at least occasionally during sex.

This is not so surprising. Fantasies are much bolder, wilder and more adventurous than everyday life. They're also tailor-made to our individual needs. In fantasy, you can have sex wherever, whenever, however, and with whomever you please! No one says they won't and no one says you can't. Fantasies allow the acting out of secret desires in the safety and privacy of the mind, with no fear or reproach.

American writer Nancy Friday, in her books on men's sexual fantasies (*Men in Love*) and women's (*My Secret Garden*), shows just how far fantasy behaviour is removed from behaviour in the Real World. In their make-believe, women have sex with complete strangers, members of their family, other women, or several men at once; men with prostitutes, virgins or several women at once. The fantasies of both sexes regularly feature rape, violence and degradation.

Because fantasies express the forbidden, they may be very exciting, but they can also be very worrying. We're afraid that our more florid fantasies will betray what we're really like underneath. What if, in an uncontrolled moment, they were to leave the mind's murky depths and come up to the surface demanding to be acted out? If a woman imagines that she's making love to another woman, does that mean she's lesbian? If a man's fantasies involve violence does that mean he's a closet Jack the Ripper or Boston Strangler? Probably not. We dream about all sorts of things — like robbing a bank, wiping out our enemies, taking over the boss's job — but we don't act them out.

Fantasies perform a valuable function. Most of us, most of the time, behave quite conservatively, sexually and otherwise. Our erotic experiences represent only the tip of the iceberg in terms of possibilities. Many possibilities only see the light of day through fantasies or dreams, seldom as reality. In the daily drama of the mind, we can identify three main actors: the Child, a primitive, pleasure-seeking, selfish character who does his best to do whatever he pleases; the Policeman, who tries to enforce law and order according to the social rules; and the Adult who does his best to keep the peace between the two. This is a huge strain on the Adult, and dreams, fantasies and jokes give him a well-earned break. In the world of make-believe, in dreams and fantasies, the Child can indulge himself down in the dungeons of the mind while the Policeman is satisfied that everything on the surface seems law-abiding enough.

Fantasies help to bridge the gap between our hidden urges and the way we're expected to behave. They are the safety valve of a normal healthy mind. They allow us to express thoughts which, if put into practice, would scandalize civilized society. They help us to strike a balance between what is possible and what is permissible.

Nor are flights of fantasy which momentarily take you away from the live partner in your arms hidden acts of unfaithfulness. They're an extension of your sexual pleasure with that person, not a substitute for that person. Should you talk about your fantasies? Some liberal souls do, and even manage to ginger up their sex lives by acting them out, which is fine if the fantasy is shared, thought there could be logistical problems if both partners' fantasy was to be raped or to have sex with same-sex partners. Nancy Friday sounds a warning note here. She recalls when she was in bed with an apparently open-minded lover, indulging in a fantasy about an anonymous lover at a football match.

'"Tell me what you're thinking" he said. I told him what I'd been thinking. He got out of bed, put on his trousers and went home.'

What bothers people most is the idea of an unknown and unseen sexual rival ('He's just using me', 'She thinks I'm a rotten lover', 'I'm not attractive enough'). If you feel there's enough trust and understanding between you, then by all means talk about your make-believe world, but bear in mind that telling your partner that, mentally, you've just been making love to half a dozen prostitutes or to the lead singer in your favourite group could go down like a lead balloon. If you have difficulty keeping your mind where your body is, it may be better to keep quiet.

TELLING YOUR PARTNER THAT YOU'VE BEEN FANTASISING ABOUT MAKING LOVE TO YOUR FAVOURITE POP STAR MIGHT NOT GO DOWN TOO WELL.

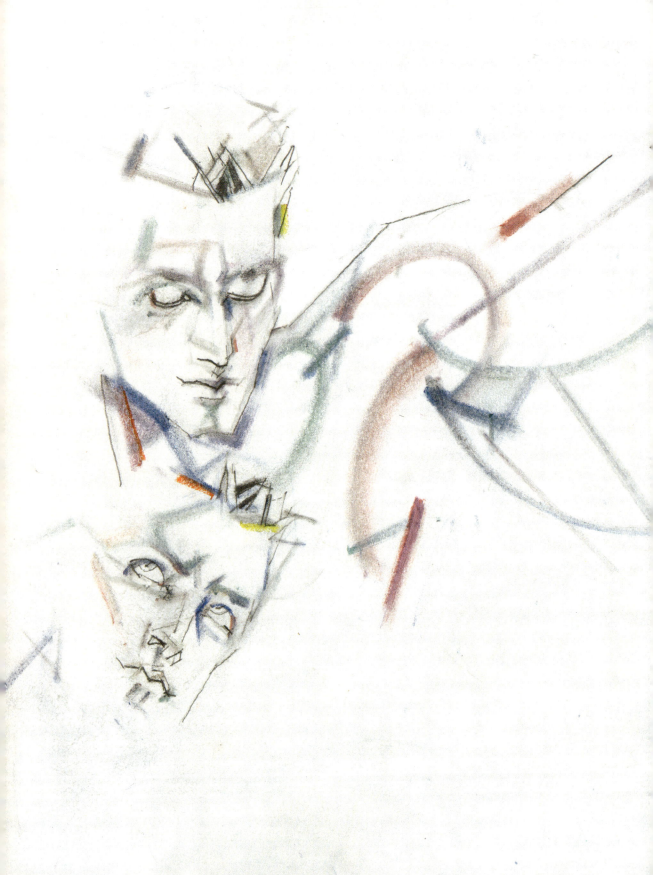

Same-sex sex

Homosexuality is the formal term used to describe sexual relationships between people of the same sex. The name comes from the Greek 'homo' meaning the same, and not the Latin 'homo' meaning man, and is applicable to both sexes. More commonly, homosexual men and women are called 'gay' and heterosexuals 'straight'.

In fact these neatly labelled boxes are by no means watertight. None of us is straightforwardly and wholeheartedly 'gay' or 'straight', but one or the other to varying degrees. Homosexuality and heterosexuality are not an either/or, but opposite ends of a range or spectrum of sexual behaviours along which people can be placed. We know from surveys that perhaps one in two adults is likely to have had one or more experiences involving someone of the same sex, and that at least half of those who haven't, have felt sexually attracted to someone of their own sex. In a majority of cases the episode or attraction is a one-off affair and usually occurs in adolescence. Left to our natural instincts probably far more of us would be attracted to people of the same sex. Certainly, when people are confined to single-sex institutions (prisons, boarding schools, ships on long voyages) for extended periods of time their sexual preferences tend to bend somewhat towards what is available.

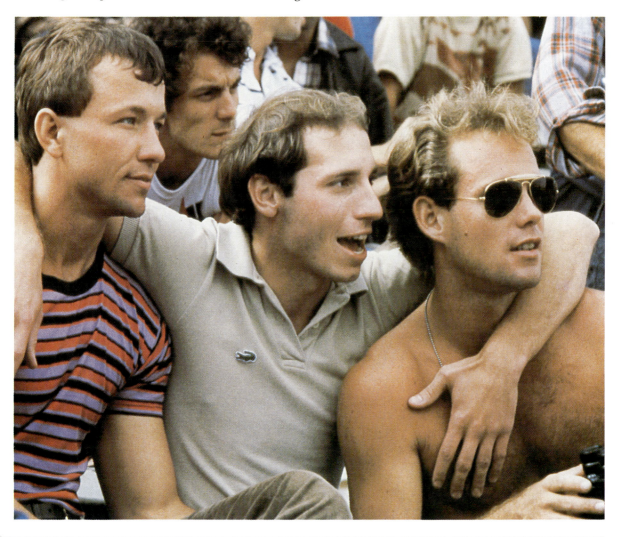

GAY RELATIONSHIPS SPAN JUST AS WIDE A SPECTRUM AS STRAIGHT RELATIONSHIPS, AND VARY FROM CASUAL ENCOUNTERS TO LONG-TERM 'MARRIAGES'.

You often hear it said that homosexuality is on the increase in our society. Certainly it is more *visible,* and visibility has a lot to do with how tolerant people's attitudes are generally. In societies where homosexuality is accepted, it will be open and public, but where it is regarded as a perversion, it will be forced underground. The fact is that there has been no society, and no time in history, when homosexuality has not existed. It occurs among very primitive peoples and in advanced societies. In ancient Greece and Rome, for example, male homosexuality was open, accepted and common, and held to be a very pure and high form of love.

In our society, it is estimated that one in ten people is fairly exclusively gay, but the number of gay women is probably smaller than the number of gay men (one of the reasons being that many women — whatever their sexual preferences — have traditionally been more financially dependent on men and therefore obliged to marry or at least cohabit with them).

British attitudes towards homosexuality have relaxed considerably over the past century. Even so, until the Wolfenden Report in 1967 and the Act of Parliament which followed it, sexual relations between men were actually a crime, and still are if either party involved is under the age of 21 (the law is silent on female homosexuality). Homosexuality was then redefined as an illness: gays were not bad, but mad, and it was up to psychologists and the medical profession to put right what was wrong. We've moved on again since then. It's now recognized that people who prefer same-sex sex are not at all ill, physically or mentally. They're perfectly happy to be the way they are, hence the term 'gay'. But members of the 'straight' community still have mixed feelings on the subject, mostly, it must be said, because they fear to examine their own same-sex impulses.

Homosexuality is still stuck with some of the old labels — 'not natural', 'against Nature' — though these are slowly fading. The taboo against homosexuality is really the old 'sex equals reproduction' idea in disguise (same-sex couples cannot possibly produce children so sex between them is wrong). But as we've already seen, sex isn't just for having babies. For anyone who fairly exclusively prefers lovers of the same sex, it's sex with the opposite sex that feels unnatural.

No one knows exactly why some people develop stronger sexual feelings for their own rather than the opposite gender. Psychologists have toyed with the theory that gay men are more likely to have had dominant mothers and weak or absent fathers, and that gay women are more likely to have had ineffectual mothers and domineering fathers, but there are plenty of heterosexual men and women who fall into these categories too. Anatomists have tried hard but unsuccessfully to prove that the pelvises of gay men are different from those of straight men. Endocrinologists have equally unsuccessfully tried to put homosexual behaviour down to hormones. What is clear is that gay people of either sex don't just *choose* to be gay (any more that non-gays choose to be heterosexual). They may choose *not* to be, by concealing their sexual orientation, some to the point of entering into heterosexual marriages, but the results are usually disastrous and short-lived. Far better to accept one's sexual identity than take on one which feels uncomfortable and is difficult to keep up.

As social prejudices have fallen away, so have many of the myths surrounding gay sexual behaviour. Homosexual men have had a reputation for having more partners than heterosexual men, and for changing them more often. In reality, gay relationships span just as wide a spectrum as straight relationships. Some gays prefer casual relationships and a lot of variety (though the spectre of AIDS has been a powerful deterrent to this kind of lifestyle), while others live in stable long-term 'marriages'.

Slowly, some of the stereotypes associated with gays are being worn down. Gay men are not typically anything, and certainly not typically effeminate, limp-wristed and lisping, any more than gay women are typically butch and masculine. These images are caricatures and now widely recognized as such.

Coming out

What does it mean? Jeffrey Weeks, author of the book *Coming Out,* explains the process as involving being open about one's sexuality, rejecting shame and guilt and an enforced 'double life,' and asserting pride in one's sexual identity. He identifies three stages in coming out:

- **Coming out to yourself,** recognising your own homosexual personality and needs.
- **Coming out to other homosexuals** and expressing sexual needs in the gay community and in relationships.
- **Coming out to other people,** declaring your sexual identity to all — perhaps the most crucial stage.

Some gays like to come out openly and publicly, complete with personal identifiers like badges; others prefer the quieter approach. But most people will feel a need to talk through their position with someone else who is gay, which invariably means enlisting support from an agency set up to offer help, like the ones listed under Useful Addresses on page 186). If the agencies themselves can't offer direct help, they will point you towards another organisation which can.

Discovering that they are homosexual comes as a shock to most people. Developing a tolerance towards different types of sexual expression is one thing, but realising that you are only going to live happily if you adopt a gay sexual identity may be quite another. So coming out may be difficult, but compared with the huge burden of living with a false identity, the relief of shaking it off can be very liberating.

Bisexuality

Some people don't feel they can easily label themselves as either heterosexual *or* homosexual; they may enjoy sexual relationships with both men and women. Sexuality is an ever-changing thing, there's no once and forever decision to be made. You may only find that you have bisexual tendencies after years of more orthodox relationships. But it's more important to recognize and accept flexibility than it is to hold onto a sexual identity that you don't feel comfortable with.

FOR MANY GAY PEOPLE, 'COMING OUT' CAN BE A DIFFICULT — BUT VERY LIBERATING — EXPERIENCE.

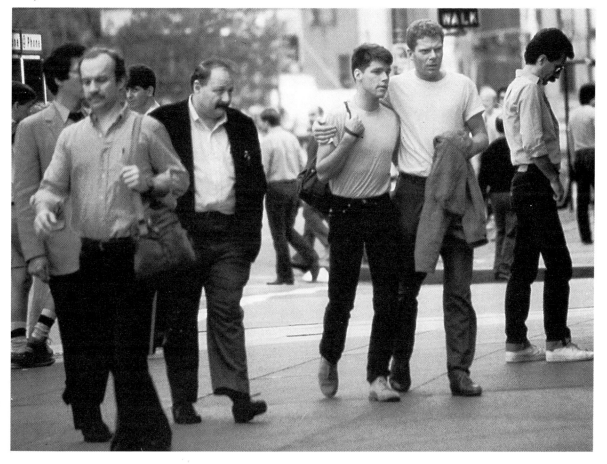

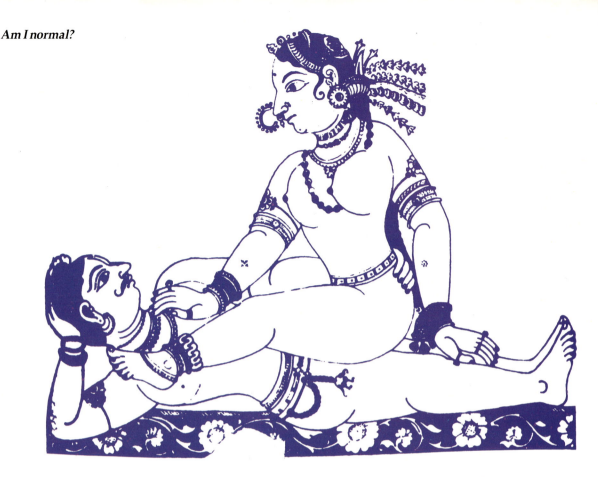

Can we try number 238?

There are quite literally hundreds of positions in which lovemaking is possible, and almost as many manuals extolling the virtues of some or other of them. The *Kama Sutra*, for example, the great Indian classic of the art of lovemaking, describes such picturesque positions as 'The Flower in Bloom', 'The Congress of the Cow' and 'Splitting Bamboo'. Many of these differ so slightly — by the angle of a fingertip or a toe, for example — that you wonder if they make any difference. Others are so complicated that passion would probably have evaporated before you got into them. And some are frankly too contorted for all but an Olympic gymnast.

You can enjoy intercourse standing up, sitting down, bending down, or on all fours, but the basic and most common position is the 'missionary' position — face to face, man on top of the woman, woman with one leg either side of the man's legs. The position gained its name when European missionaries introduced it to natives with more eclectic tastes who were amazed to find a group of people who stuck to one position!

The obvious advantages of the missionary position are that the lovers can see and talk to each other more easily, but it is a somewhat awkward position in which to directly stimulate the woman's clitoris — many, if not

most, women need to have their clitoris stimulated to reach a climax. Some women find the man's pubic bone pressing on the clitoris or the tugging of the penis on the lips of the vulva does the trick, but it's quite difficult for the penis alone to stimulate the clitoris. As Bernie Zilbergeld says in his book *Men and Sex*, '...you need an L-shaped penis and you don't see many of them any more'. The missionary position isn't very good for anorexic ladies with heavyweight partners either. Nor does it allow the penis to penetrate very deeply, unless the woman puts a cushion under her bottom or raises her legs by bending her knees up or hooking her heels over her partner's shoulders.

Preferable from all these standpoints might be the positions in which the woman sits astride the man while he is on his back (though there may be some men who feel sensitive about having the woman in a superior position). This gives more scope for stimulation of the clitoris, either by the man or the woman herself. The same can be said for positions in which the man inserts his penis from behind. 'Rear entry' positions are the nearest we get to the way in which animals couple, which is why they offend some people. Yet humans are the only higher animals to make love face to face; they also have more imagination

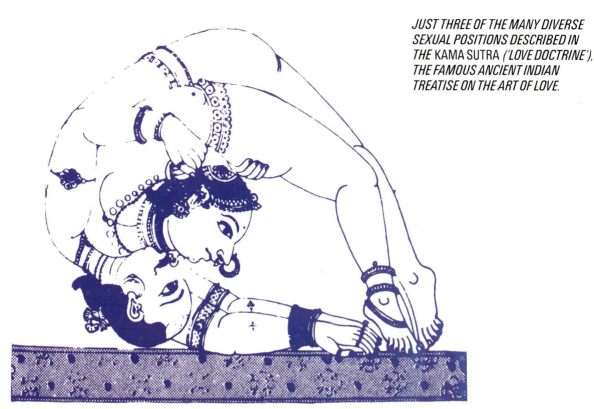

JUST THREE OF THE MANY DIVERSE SEXUAL POSITIONS DESCRIBED IN THE KAMA SUTRA *('LOVE DOCTRINE'), THE FAMOUS ANCIENT INDIAN TREATISE ON THE ART OF LOVE.*

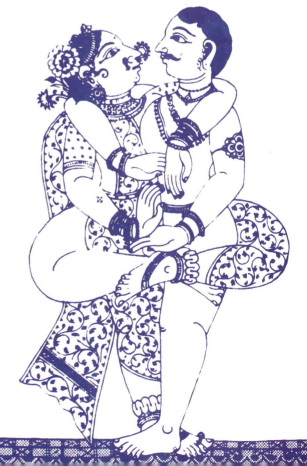

and curiosity than animals so it's not surprising they want to make love in different positions. Several basic positions allow rear entry: the woman can kneel forward on her elbows and knees (the 'doggy' position), both partners can lie on their sides, with the man behind (the 'spoons' position), or the woman can lie face down with her legs apart on the edge of the bed, while the man grips her thighs and stands up (the 'wheelbarrow' position).

Couples tend to adopt the positions they find most comfortable and familiar, but it's quite usual at the start of a relationship or later when sexual appetites are getting a little jaded to try out a whole variety of positions. But you don't need to be a sexual gymnast to enjoy yourself. It may be *possible* to have sex swinging from a chandelier, standing on your head, or on top of Grandma's Welsh dresser, but you can't bank on it being more enjoyable or satisfying than the old standards.

Sex during menstruation

Some societies regard a woman as 'unclean' while she is menstruating. There is no medical basis for this attitude. Intercourse at this time can be messy, but a woman is unlikely to get pregnant during her period, though it is just possible. It's a matter of personal taste.

Oral sex

As children, we all use our mouths for exploring things, so why not for exploring a lover's body? Many couples find oral sex extremely satisfying and intimate. The highly sensitive and agile mouth and tongue can lick and probe more subtly and delicately than fingertips and provide more interesting sensations. Also, many men and women find the close-up view, and the taste and smell, of their partner's physically aroused genitals very exciting.

Slang idiom for oral sex includes 'going down on someone' and 'having a blow job' (though in fact there's no blowing involved). More formally, oral sex is given two Latin tags: *cunnilingus*, when the man licks and sucks the woman's clitoris and vagina, and *fellatio*, when the woman does the same to the man's penis and testes. When both partners want to lick each other at the same time, they often adopt a position where each is coiled head to tail, hence the term 'soixante-neuf' or 69.

Given early childhood taboos it's not surprising that many people are afraid their natural secretions will be offensive or distasteful to a partner. Obviously, careful attention to hygiene (more on this in Chapter 12) is essential, but the fluids of a fresh clean vagina can have a powerfully arousing effect on a man. So can the taste of semen for a woman. Swallowing semen is absolutely harmless and might even have some nutritional value (the average teaspoonful contains, as well as protein in the sperm, the sugar fructose, ascorbic acid, small amounts of zinc and traces of cholesterol, and has the calorific value of raw carrot!).

Sexploitation

Any sexual act which takes place without the consent of one of the participants is wrong. For one person to be forced cajoled, bribed, threatened or in any other way persuaded to have sex against their will is totally unacceptable. Unfortunately, though, there are many situations in which it is difficult to say no. It may be that one person has power over another by virtue of their age, their superior physical strength, their authority or status. But in every case it means that people are being treated as possessions instead of individuals — which is likely to cause pain, humiliation and guilt.

In most countries the victims of unwelcome sexual advances are protected by law. Thus in Britain any act of sex with a minor or a mentally defective person is against the law, as is sex between members of the same family and with a woman without her consent.

The problem is that all these crimes are notoriously under-reported. Sexually abused children find it difficult to tell on a loved parent or a feared adult. Rape victims and those who have suffered sexual harassment worry, often justifiably, that they might not be believed and that the resultant publicity might do them more harm than good.

Yet victims of sexual exploitation *do* need to talk. This is partly because frightened and confused feelings need to be worked through if they are going to be prevented from permanently marring future relationships and feelings of self-esteem; and partly because reporting an incident is one way of putting a stop to it. If you find yourself in a position of being exploited sexually and you have no one to talk to, you should contact one of the specialist help agencies listed at the back of the book, under Useful Addresses.

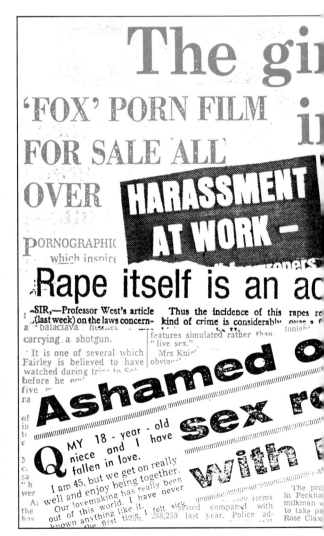

Variety with responsibility_____

There are probably as many ways of making love as there are lovers. Some like bright light on the subject, others like to hide in the dark. Some prefer open fields, others insist on a comfy bed. Some like to be deadly serious, others like to giggle. Some like to talk and shout, others like to keep quiet. But whatever you like, in sex as in most things, there is nothing new under the sun. Most preferences and positions and places have been tried out by someone, somewhere.

Whatever you decide to do together, or separately, whether you opt for routine or variety, and no matter what variants or accessories you choose, there are some basic rules.

■ **Don't do anything you don't enjoy.** You can enjoy someone else's pleasure or you can enjoy your own, but enjoyment must be there somewhere.

■ **Don't do anything that will hurt or injure feelings or bodies,** yours, your partner's or anyone else's. This requires a considerable amount of thought and a great deal of responsibility.

■ **Don't do something to someone else that you wouldn't like that person to do to you,** and contrariwise don't ask that person to do for you what you are not prepared to do for him or her.

Observe these basics: sex is all about sharing pleasures and taking care of feelings.

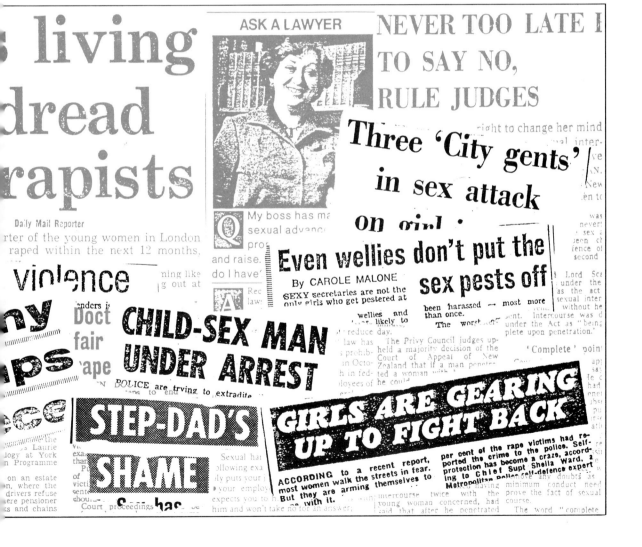

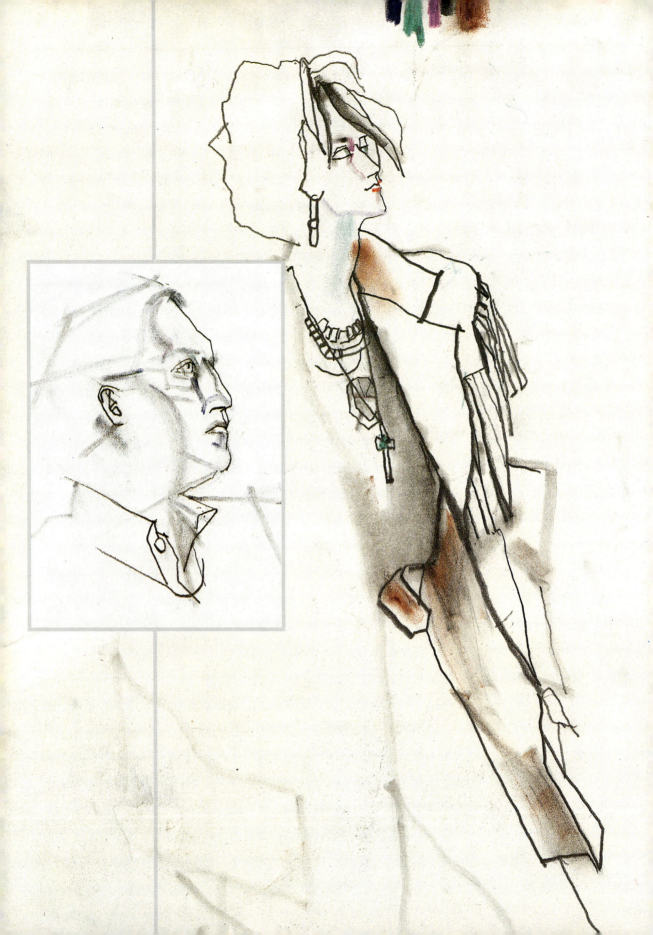

9 Lopsided liaisons

The path of true love is not always straight even in ideal circumstances. We don't choose our partners so much as fall for them, sometimes against our better judgement, and there can be disparities between ourselves and those we love which actually work against the relationship. It's not so much a question of our own attitudes to differences in age, or class, or religion, or race, so much as other people's attitudes to these things. After all, it is other people who create the climate we live in. This doesn't mean that relationships with inbuilt discrepancies are doomed, just that we need to embark on them with our eyes open rather than tight shut.

Age gaps

In our society the usual pattern has been for women to go out and eventually settle down, with men who are a couple of years older than they are. The reasons conventionally put forward for this are that girls tend to mature earlier than boys, so boys of equivalent maturity tend to be at least a couple of years older. There's also a widespread assumption that women choose men according to their ability to provide financial security, which tends to increase as the man gets older, while men choose women according to their ability to produce children, which is more likely the younger the woman is.

Actually, when you consider that women are becoming more and more able to provide for themselves, and that they live on average eight years longer than men *and* that they don't reach their sexual peak until their mid-thirties (men do so in their early twenties), it might be a more sensible arrangement if men married older women!

Of course we rarely go through such calculations when we fall in love. There is no ideal age gap between people who like each other. In general, we choose partners of the same generation as ourselves, give or take a year or two, because we tend to communicate more easily with them. Although in later life age differences melt away into nothing, in our teens and early twenties even one year makes a big difference. We think of people only a year or two older than ourselves as has-beens and those a year or two younger as babes in arms!

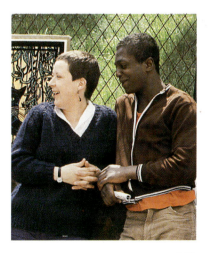

> '*I was 20 and he was 19. I was a bit self-conscious at first. Friends teased me and said I was cradle-snatching! But he acts a lot older than me, so it's OK isn't it?*' MANDY

'I was 26 and he was 20...Aren't you going to comment on that? Most people do.' JENNY

Traditionally men who 'date down' are frowned on less than women who do the same, perhaps for biological reasons — a man is capable of fathering children long after a woman's childbearing years are over. Even so older man/younger woman relationships can provoke comments like 'He's old enough to be her father!'.

Some men find the answer to their mid-life crisis in a fling with someone younger — a younger woman is living proof that they're not heading towards their dotage. And to some young women, a man ten or even twenty years their senior stands for emotional security, wisdom and, in more than a few cases, money.

'I was bored with men of my own age. All they do is take a girl out and then brag about her among themselves. You're forever competing for time with the lads who want to go out for a drink. I didn't feel special. With Mike it's different, he's been through all the business of proving he's good sexually. He wants to travel, go to the theatre, do things. I feel far more relaxed with him.' AMANDA

Funnily enough, men on the receiving end of an older woman's affections often feel more secure, despite the occasional raised eyebrow, than the women who love them. One study revealed that twice as many men were prepared to admit to having been in love with an older woman than women would admit to having been in love with a younger man. The numbers clearly don't add up, so unless a lot of younger men were being loved by the same older woman, someone wasn't telling the truth!

Sometimes we seek out partners older or younger than ourselves as a way of coping with insecurity. A woman may be looking for someone to take care of her, a replacement father in effect, or she may not feel confident enough to compete with women of her own age. Men who 'date down' sometimes do so because their egos cannot handle being faced with an emotionally or intellectually superior partner, which women of their own age or older may seem to be.

Problems of a darker nature may surface if one partner is stuck in the child-parent groove. A younger man or woman who, to begin with, seeks security from an older partner may come to resent his or her dependence as the relationship progresses and there seems to be no room to grow up. An older man who is attracted to a younger woman, because her dependence and hero worship of him puffs him up, can become addicted to these things; as she tries to grow, he feels threatened, and deep cracks may appear in the relationship. Similarly a younger man/older woman relationship may break up when the man discovers that the relationship has given him the sexual security he lacked when he felt he was unable to compete for younger women.

Really, the answer is 'Go ahead', provided you and your partner are also compatible in ways which have nothing to do with age.

'There's nearly nine years between us and we've been together for three. We clicked emotionally from the moment we met — we sense each other's moods very quickly. He's tremendously good with people, very gentle but very persistent. He thinks I'm good with people too. We both like feelings, talking about feelings, our own and other people's. Neither of us likes rules. We're always doing things on the spur of the moment. When I think of some of the boyfriends I had before him! They were so wooden and unadventurous!' CLEO

THERE'S NO IDEAL AGE GAP BETWEEN PEOPLE WHO ARE IN LOVE WITH ONE ANOTHER — EVEN THOUGH YOUNG PEOPLE TEND TO THINK OF THOSE ONLY A YEAR OR TWO OLDER THAN THEMSELVES AS HAS-BEENS!

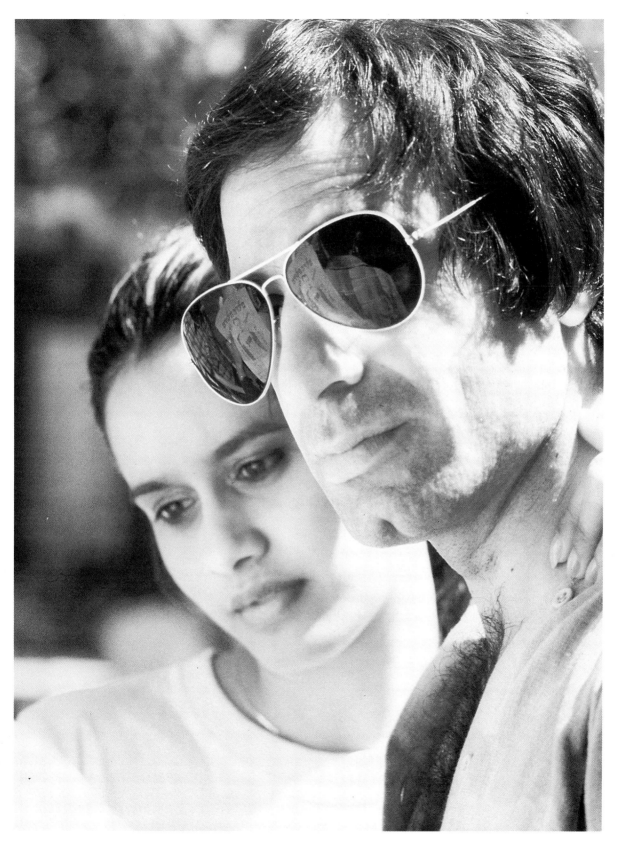

Mixing married and singles_____

The prospects of a married/single relationship leading anywhere satisfying are a good deal less than fifty-fifty. It may suit some people to be in a relationship where there's no promise of commitment, but for the vast majority it's likely to be full of problems, especially for the single partner, and for the partner of the married man or woman.

What makes married people seek out singles? — that tends to be the pattern, not the other way round. How can you tell whether it's a fling or something more serious? Some people claim they have an 'open marriage', one which allows them extramarital freedom. This should be taken with a pinch of salt. Very, very few couples manage such arrangements. It's more likely that both partners have decided there's not much left in their marriage but don't feel quite ready to end it, so they play the field to see if the grass really is greener outside marriage. The old loose emotional ends haven't yet been tied up but both partners feel the need to form new relationships. More usually 'open marriage' is a misnomer for a marriage in which one partner has itchy feet and the other tolerates infidelity rather than lose the straying partner altogether. Even if spouses agree to give each other extramarital freedom, the practice often blows the theory — jealousy has little regard for thoughts worked out in the head and can quickly put paid to any tidy pacts. If you are very attracted to someone who is married, what are the problems you are likely to face? Here are a few of the commonest.

■ **Have you given any thought to your loved one's other partner?** Just how honest are you all being with each other? Does his/her wife/husband know? Are there children involved?

■ **You'll probably feel very lonely at times,** unless you have plenty of other friends. You'll miss your mate most at holiday times and at weekends, times when he or she is expected to be with the family and cannot join you. Lonely feelings will become more acute when you realize that you may, permanently, be expected to take second place.

■ **You may be restricted in the number of friends you can share,** even the number of friends you can tell if it's a clandestine affair. This can put a strain on both of you and limit your social life.

■ **The cards are stacked against your relationship.** All the social supports — a home, a family, public approval, legal status — are with the married partner, not the single one. Your married lover is going to find it far more difficult to get out of his or her marriage than out of the relationship with you.

■ **Married lovers seldom leave their spouses.** They may swear blue in the face they will, but get cold feet when it comes to the crunch. At the eleventh hour they may realize that every relationship has its problems, so what guarantee is there that a relationship with you will be different?

■ **Relationships between married and singles often suffer from having nowhere to go,** not just literally in the sense of finding the time and the place to meet, but in the sense of making plans, of carving out a path together through life, or fulfilling some of the goals and expectations talked about in the next chapter.

Let's suppose that a marriage really *is* on its last legs, and that there is a prospect of happiness with a new partner. Both of you should be aware that there may be a lot of left-over feelings which need to be worked through. The deserted partner rarely gives up without a struggle and there are often children, property, possessions and painful feelings to sort out. In general, it's best to tie up all the loose ends, even if it takes a year or two, before rushing headlong into a new relationship. It's not really fair to load a new partner with a lot of practical problems, as well as resentments and grudges.

So the essential ingredient in any survival strategy for mixing marrieds and singles is realism. Go into the whole thing with your eyes wide open. Don't take as gospel stories along the lines of 'My spouse doesn't understand me/support me/appreciate me/have sex with me', and then ask yourself if things would be so very different between the two of you.

MIXED MATCHES HAVE A LOT TO OFFER — BUT THEY NEED SOME EXTRA THOUGHT TO MAKE THEM WORK.

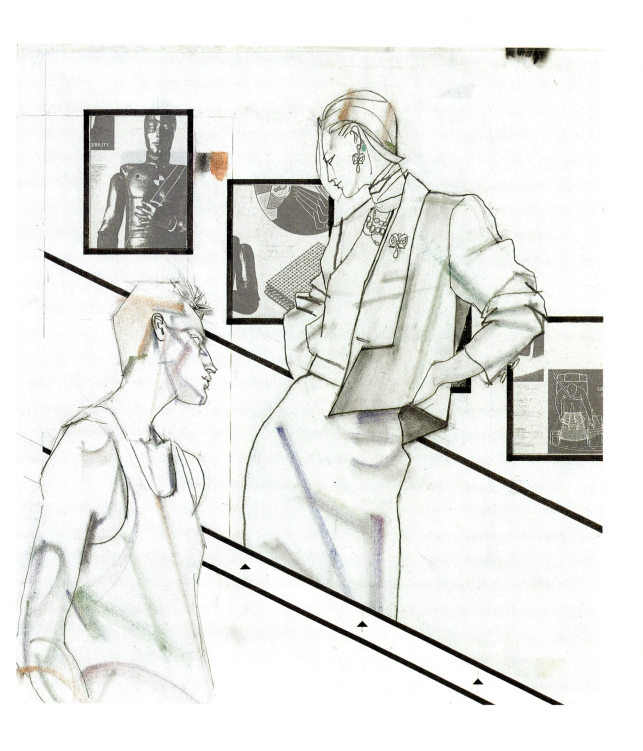

The class dimension

In the last half century class differences have not disappeared, but they have become subtler and more complex. In the old days, people from the top drawer were also blessed with money, power and education, while the humbly born had none of these things. But in dozens of small ways, class differences still make themselves felt — in the way we eat and speak, in our attitudes towards law and order, towards domestic arrangements, towards money, towards clothes and furniture and cars — all those things that crafty advertisers play upon. People can still be very snobbish if they think that one of their friends or a member of their family is going out with someone 'beneath' them or, by the same sentiment inverted, with someone who is a 'toff'. Here is how one young man described the traumas of a relationship which, happily, turned into a very stable marriage.

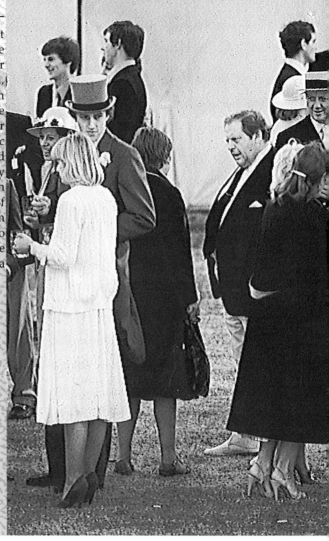

'Julia was definitely ashamed of my broad accent. She was actually very much in love with me and I could tell she was desperately trying to overcome her old dyed-in-the-wool prejudices — inherited from her family. But she found it very difficult. She didn't introduce me to her friends for a long time and when she did I found out they'd been under the impression she'd been going out with a married man! Imagine…she actually preferred to live with that stigma rather than admit to going out with someone of a lower social class! I found that very upsetting. What upset me even more was her mother's reaction. When we finally decided to get married, her family were reluctant to invite any of my side to the wedding. Half of them couldn't have afforded to hire topper and tails anyway. To add insult to injury, her mother insisted that I went to elocution lessons. I'm ashamed to say I did. I wouldn't dream of doing such a thing now. I think more of myself. I'd tell her where to get off!' PAUL

We tend to think more highly of people if they share our values. Mix with people whose values are different and life can get rather uncomfortable. If your family and friends think money and possessions are important they won't be impressed by a studious boyfriend who's scratching around for funds to complete his doctorate. If they rate education highly they'll be pretty frosty towards the supermarket check-out girl who left school at 16. Finding a social environment in which you and your partner both feel comfortable may mean giving up some of your sniffier friends, but maybe they weren't worth having in the first place.

Far harder to come to terms with are your own reactions towards differences between yourself and your partner. When the first flush of excitement cools, you may find yourself getting irritated by things you never thought you were small-minded enough to care about, like the way he balances peas on his fork/smothers everything with ketchup/says 'pardon' or 'pleased to meet you', or the way she says 'orf' rather than 'off'/insists on Pimms and pickled walnuts/snorts when she laughs. Even if quirks like this are just about bearable when you're alone together, they may blow up out of all proportion when you're in company. Are you sure it's other people doing the noticing and minding? Or does the presence of other people serve to bring your own prejudices flooding to the surface? It's important to do some soul-searching before tensions like these mar your relationship irreparably.

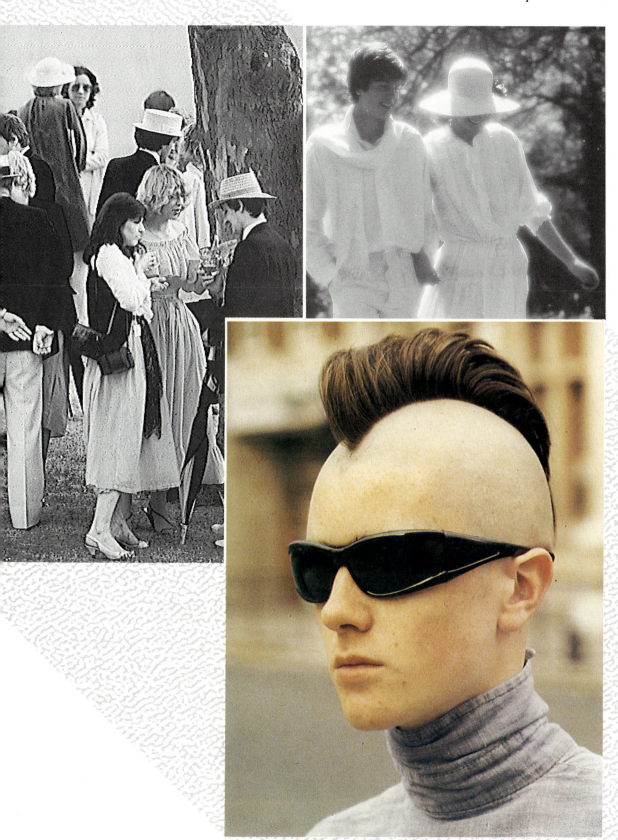

Religious beliefs

It may not occur to you to think of religious differences as a problem area. Britain is not a deeply religious society; only one in seven people attends church regularly, only one in three brides is married in church, and fewer than half the babies born in Britain are baptized. Nevertheless the faith we are born in can exert its influence in subtler ways. If your partner is Catholic, for example, he or she may have views on contraception which no amount of reasoning on your part will shake. If one of you is Jewish there may be friction over whether your son, when the time comes, should be circumcised.

And if you decide to give up your faith to avoid problems between you and your partner, your family might not approve. If you decide, for example, to forego a religious wedding and settle for a Registry Office ceremony instead, be prepared for strong feelings and hurt reactions from your parents and family. It helps to anticipate and discuss likely reactions with your partner and decide how to deal with them. If you have a joint strategy you're less likely to fall out with each over even if you cross swords with others.

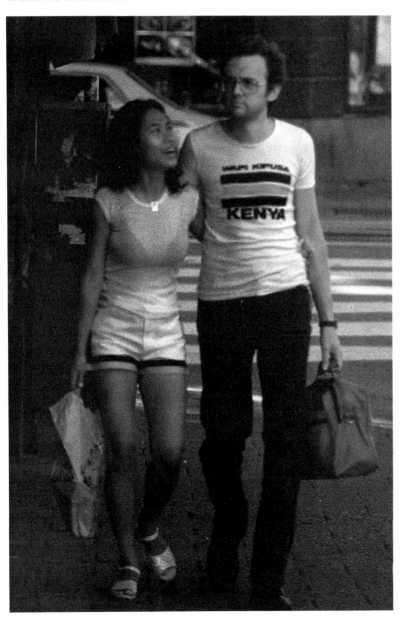

THE MORE INTER-RACIAL RELATIONSHIPS THERE ARE . . .

. . . THE LESS OUT OF THE ORDINARY THEY WILL BE SEEN TO BE.

Racial origins

Judging by the marriage statistics, partnerships between people with different ethnic roots are far less common than partnerships between people of different faiths. While about 50 per cent of Protestant and Roman Catholic marriages performed today and 40 per cent of Jewish marriages involve people of different creeds, fewer than 1 per cent of all marriages is truly inter-racial.

It's perhaps not surprising that so few actually make it to the altar. Inter-race relationships are not doomed to failure but there is a certain amount of adjustment to be made. The charming Greek or Italian who manages to find just enough English to tell you how wonderful you are may have a certain exotic appeal…until he spirits you back to his native land and you find it considerably more male-dominated than your own liberal environment. Women particularly face problems of

adjustment when they fall in love with men from cultures which place all sorts of restrictions on women's freedom. Your partner may be tolerant enough, but will that tolerance survive the entrenched attitudes all around you?

The problems multiply when there are very obvious differences between you, such as the colour of your skin. None of your friends may bat an eyelid, but ignorance and a primitive fear of 'foreigners' can bring out a most unpleasant vein of cruelty in strangers. The fact that this *shouldn't* be so is no reason for kidding yourselves that it won't be so. Yet the more inter-racial relationships there are, the less out-of-the-ordinary they will be seen to be. That may be little consolation if you're the object of hostile reactions now, but it might help a little to think that you could be paving the way for greater tolerance eventually.

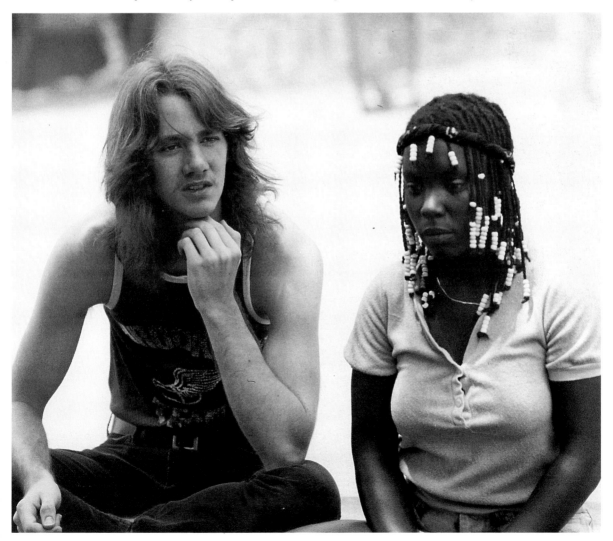

Mixing colour and creed _____

Once upon a time — and not so long ago either — the boundaries between social and cultural groups were so deeply etched that they might have been oceans, so effectively did they keep people apart. You crossed these social boundaries at your peril for you risked being ostracized by family and friends if you did.

Today, in our multiracial society, in which people move up and down the social scale and rub shoulders daily with people of many different backgrounds, the boundaries have lost some of their deterrent power. Even if we mix mostly with people of the same faith, income bracket and racial origin at school, when we get to college or go out to work we're thrown together with people from every walk of life.

Not surprisingly, young people today are far more liberal in their attitudes to dating than their parents were. In a survey of the views of 200 American teenagers, 97 per cent said that religious denomination didn't matter when they were choosing someone to go out with, and 75 per cent said they had no objection to marrying someone of a different faith.

Ideally it should be so. Differences add spice to life. Things would be very dull if we all thought, spoke, looked and acted alike. Different accents and manners hold a certain fascination for us and arouse our curiosity. It's easy to see why Lady Chatterley fell for the gamekeeper.

It would be nice to think that the old prejudices were disappearing among the older generation too, but old prejudices die hard. However well educated, sophisticated and liberal we ourselves may feel, there are some deep-rooted intolerances that can emerge to blight even the most promising relationship. Mixed matches have their difficult moments, so if you're contemplating one, it's worth familiarizing yourself with some of the obstacles around the course. Your feelings for your partner are going to have to be strong enough to withstand above average pressures.

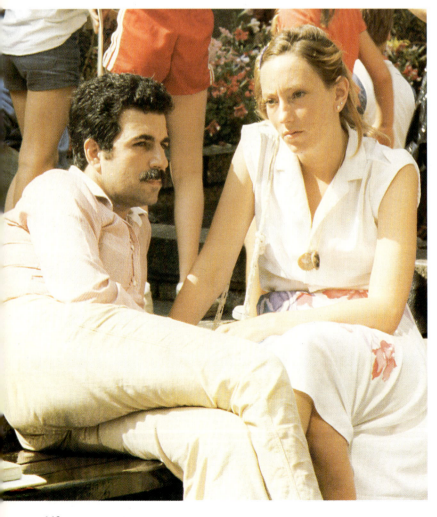

THE PATH OF TRUE LOVE NEVER RUNS SMOOTH — AND A MIXED MATCH MAY RESULT IN AN EXTRA BUMPY RIDE.

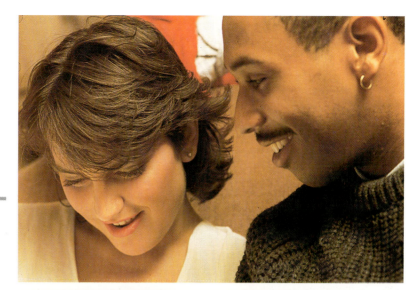

PARTNERSHIPS BETWEEN PEOPLE
WITH DIFFERENT ETHNIC ROOTS ARE
FAR LESS COMMON THAN
PARTNERSHIPS BETWEEN PEOPLE OF
DIFFERENT RELIGIOUS FAITHS.

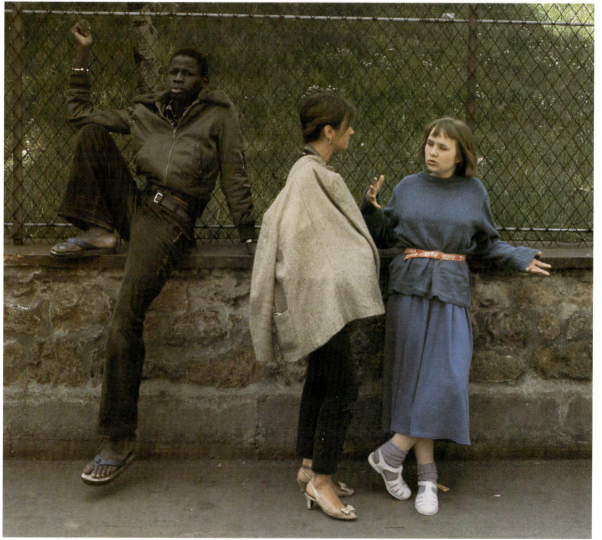

Coping with parents

Some of the most heated rows in families surround a son's or daughter's choice of friends. Having an independent social life is an obvious way of saying that your social and emotional needs are no longer satisfied within the family. Nevertheless we need love and support from our parents — they're difficult commodities to do without. Who you choose as friends will very much determine how much of a foot you can keep in the parental door.

Rows about spending money, the way you look, the state of your room and so on punctuate most family environments. Then you start going out with someone your parents don't approve of; he or she is too old/too young/too stand-offish/too rough…and everything changes. Suddenly the rules get tightened up; you're expected to go out less often, come in earlier and say where you're going.

Try to see it their way. What seems like a harmless romance to you looks like a horror movie to them. *You* may have no intention of a permanent relationship but *they're* looking to the future and imagining spending high days and holidays in the company of someone they have nothing in common with. Worse, they may think this person is going to ruin all their well-laid plans for you. If they've skimped and saved to give their daughter a good education, her passion for a

HGV driver will *not* please them; if they're proud of their working class roots, their son's affair with a stockbroker's daughter will seem like the deepest treachery; not to mention the problems of parents who see their son or daughter involved with a partner the same age as themselves.

Remember that your parents usually want the best for you. Their motives are good even if their methods seem misguided. And it really is best for everyone if you can stay on good terms with them.

So give them a good hearing. Find out why they think your friend is not right for you. Ask yourself whether their fears just might be well-founded. At the same time explain your own views. If you feel theirs are bigoted and narrow-minded, say so. If you feel offended that they don't trust you to look after yourself, then say that too. But do so in a way that shows you want to avoid confrontation if at all possible and aim for compromise.

You can point out that you don't intend to settle down for life with this person (if you don't) but that you are enjoying his or her company. Or you can point out that you *do* intend a long-term relationship (if you do) and get across to them how happy you are together and how desperately miserable you'd be apart. Few parents can deny their children contentment in life.

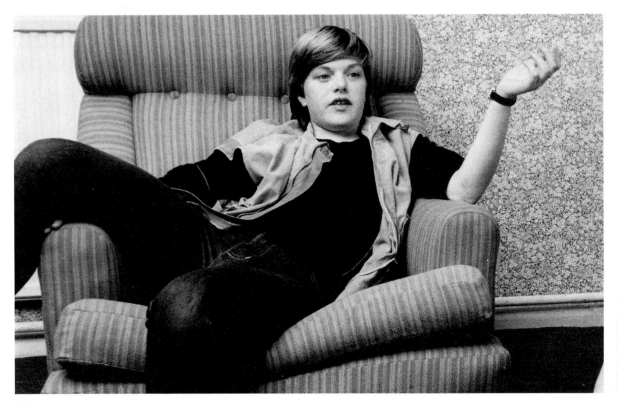

What do you do — short of acting in downright defiance — if you find yourself up against a brick wall? Probably very little, except be patient. *Giving in* to parents and *giving up* your partner is *not* the answer — you'll harbour such resentment against your parents that it will only worsen your relationship with them. The important thing is to be absolutely honest about what you're doing. If they've banned your friend from the house, tell them when and where you are seeing him or her. Hopefully, they will respect your openness. It is, after all, your life.

WHETHER YOU'RE ON GOOD TERMS WITH YOUR PARENTS WILL OFTEN DEPEND ON WHO YOU CHOOSE AS YOUR FRIENDS.

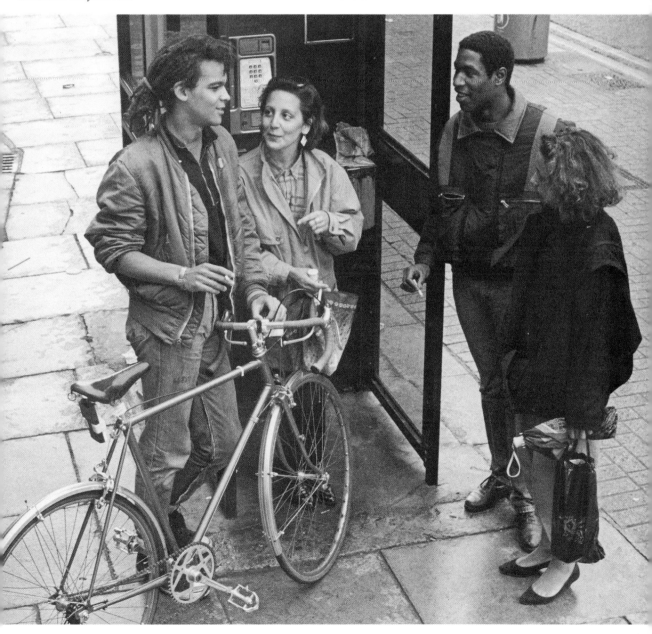

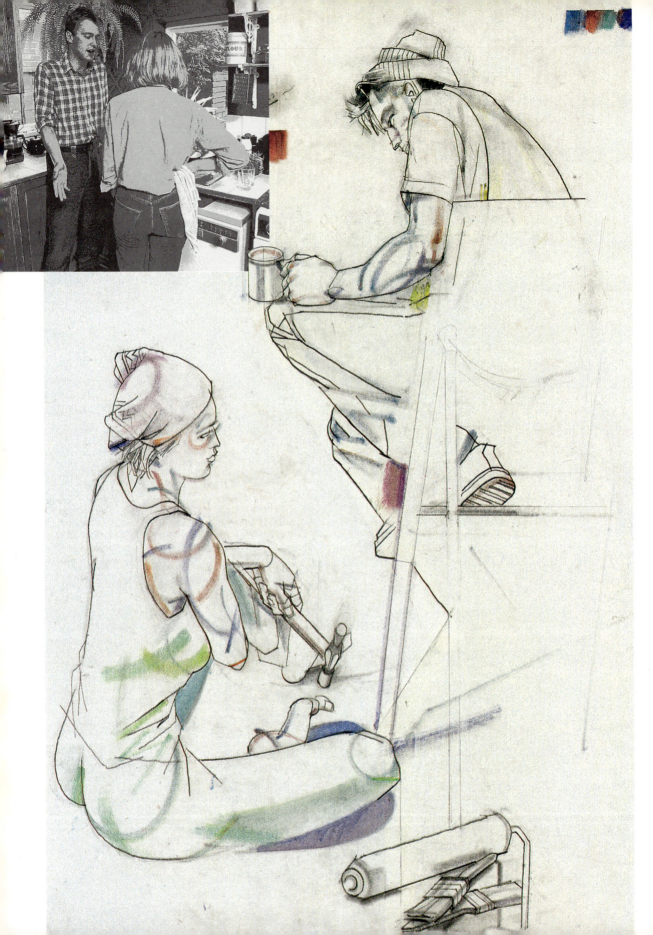

10
Till death do us part

More and more couples today are setting up home without marrying. Some eventually do 'make it legal'. In fact, the increase in the number of 'paper marriages', as the Danes call them, is probably one of the most dramatic social changes of recent years. British studies show that in 1980 one in five couples lived together before getting married, compared with one in ten in 1975 and only one in thirty in 1970. Why is this?

Marriage versus living together

There's no sign that marriage itself is losing its popularity. Official figures show that 95 per cent of the population take the plunge before their fortieth birthday, and although divorce is on the increase, remarriage is more popular than ever before. What *is* happening is that people are marrying later. In 1980 the average British woman married at 23 (a year later than in the late 1960s) and the average British man at 25. At the same time, we're seeing far fewer teenage brides. One woman in five marrying in 1982 was under 20, compared with one in three in 1972.

We marry later because we stay at school and college longer. Girls today have career options their Victorian grandmothers never dreamed of, and are anxious to get as much job experience as they can before marriage and motherhood. They're also less likely to be catapulted into premature marriage by unplanned pregnancy. Access to good birth control methods and a more relaxed attitude towards single parents have halved the number of 'shot-gun' weddings in the past twenty years.

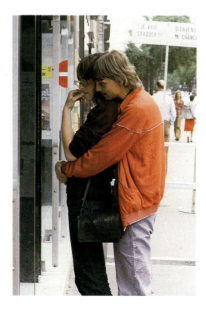

If living together is helping to delay marriage, might it not be bringing the divorce rate down too? As a rule, the earlier you marry the more likely you are to find yourself in the divorce court. More than half of teenage marriages end in divorce or separation; people marrying in their teens are twice as likely to split up as people marrying in their late twenties and three times as likely to split up as those who marry in their thirties.

The reasons for this high casualty rate are not hard to find. Psychologists say that many early marriages are triggered by panic, by the fear that the longer you leave it the less choice you'll have — not a very firm foundation for a lifelong commitment. Also, when we're in our teens we're still growing and changing emotionally. It's hard to wake up one morning and find you're with someone you hardly recognize. Married teenagers are also likely to be surrounded by unmarried friends who seem intent on showing them what a beanfeast single life is — 'the grass is greener on the other side' syndrome.

'What do I gain from living with my partner?'

If it's the blessing of the church, the state or Aunt Madge you're after, then probably not a lot. But if you're looking for flexibility, the opportunity to explore a relationship that will allow you to develop and find yourself, then living together may have some plus points.

People who live together do so because they feel the need for prolonged periods of close contact but are realistic enough to see that the relationship might be a 'now-but-not-for-ever' one. They want relationship experience without feeling hemmed in. They want to keep their options open and avoid commitments like mortgages and families just in case they feel like spreading their wings. In many ways it's more responsible to be honest about this, than to plunge into marriage vows which you fear you might break.

Obviously living together offers more intimacy than just going out together — you can be with each other in a much wider range of situations. But living together does not mean sexual freedom any more than marriage does. In fact there is evidence to suggest that couples living together are *more* likely to be faithful to each other than couples who are married. Nor is it likely to be a non-stop orgy of sexual pleasure! When you live together you have to sort out all kinds of mundane problems, like who'll do the cooking/washing/cleaning/shopping, and whether one of you can read in bed if the other wants the light off. Very romantic.

All told then, 'later rather than sooner' seems to be the golden rule for a lasting marriage. What cohabitation seems to do is postpone the wedding bells, not undermine marriage as an institution. Most people who live together plan to get married eventually, thought not necessarily to each other. Time will tell whether trial marriages will help to reduce the number of broken ones, but at least they reduce the proportion that don't even make it past the teething stage.

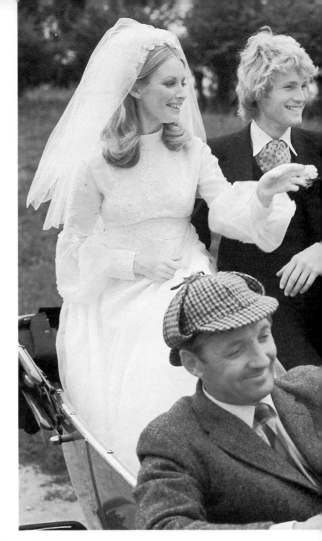

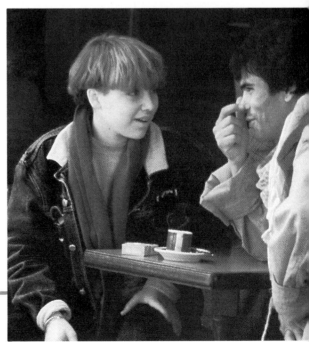

MARRIAGE VERSUS LIVING TOGETHER? ALWAYS A DIFFICULT QUESTION TO ANSWER WHEN YOU'VE DECIDED ON A LONG-TERM RELATIONSHIP.

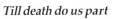

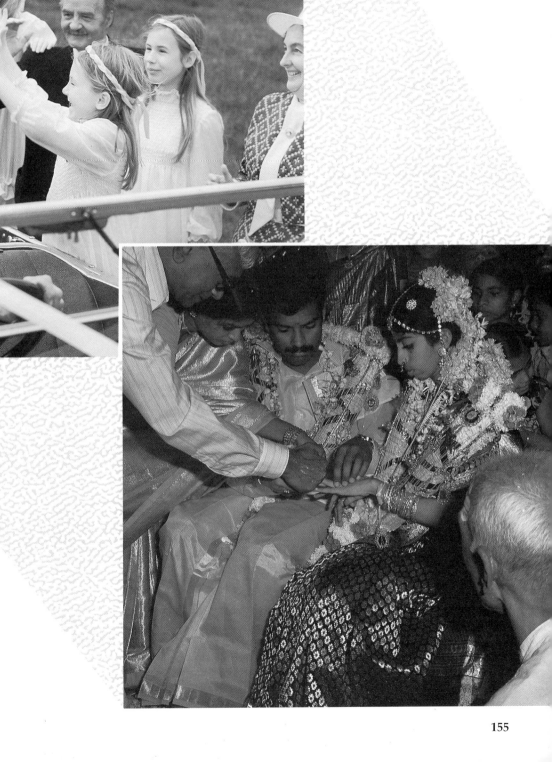

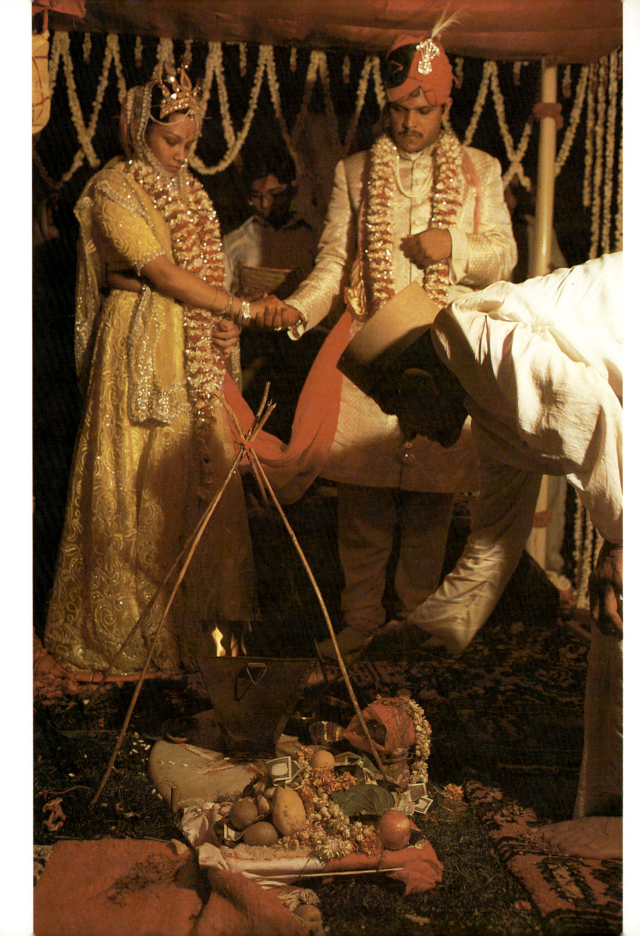

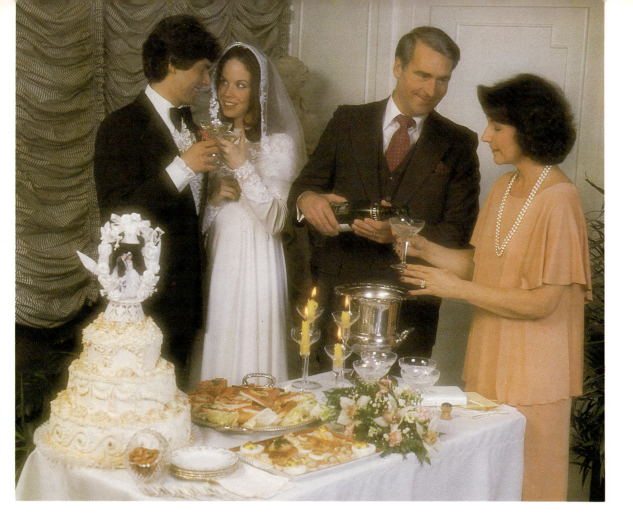

It's from these more forgettable moments in life that you'll get a good idea of whether you can muddle along together on a permanent basis. One of you may turn out to be compulsively tidy, the other completely chaotic. One of you may turn out to be obsessively secretive, the other very frank and open. One of you might thrive on an endless stream of friends, the other favour more solitary pursuits. The attraction of opposites, for all its strength in bringing you together (psychologists say we like to feel we have qualities the other person lacks, and vice versa), may be the force that eventually drives you apart. Studies of marriage show that couples who stay together tend to be more like each other than those who split up.

Living together, then, may be a good precautionary measure if you feel you need a little more self-knowledge, a little more convincing that it could be a once-and-for-always relationship. There are no copper-bottomed guarantees with marriage, but most people feel that when they marry it should at least feel as if it's for life. All relationships hurt when they break up, but if there are legal battles to go through things could be far more painful. Better to go through a trial marriage than a divorce if you're not sure.

THE MARRIAGE CEREMONY: FOR SOME AN EXPENSIVE AND OUT-OF-DATE PIECE OF RITUAL, FOR OTHERS AN ESSENTIAL ACT TO MARK THE BEGINNING OF A CHANGE IN STATUS.

Should we get married?

For some people who are living together there is no chance of marriage because they're gay or because one or the other is. For others, the decision not to take marriage vows is deliberate, a statement to the world that they don't believe in the institution. Or it may simply be a way of avoiding the pomp and ceremony of the wedding itself.

Unless any of these apply to you, there are few pointers to what is best for your individual circumstances. The decision is an essentially personal one. There are some advantages which apply to everyone. Taxes are heavier for single people, for example. But most people's reasons for marrying are not so practical:

> *We got married because it was uncomfortable when David's father, who is getting on in years, came for weekends. That's exactly how David proposed. He said 'It would make it easier with Dad if we got married'. I didn't want him to get down on his knees exactly, but all the same it wasn't very romantic.* DAWN

Granted, this *wasn't* a very romantic reason for marrying, but it's probably not such an unusual reason for those living together to make their union legal. Social pressures can be very strongly felt, and there's no underestimating the powerful effect of other people's disapproval.

There's no doubt that marriage does remove some embarrassments in coping with the outside world. If you've spent awkward weekends hiding your partner's half of the wardrobe and explaining away the double bed to visiting parents, there will be a sense of relief from being able to drop the façade.

Nor is there any doubt that there is something comforting about customs and ritual. Getting married, for those who choose to do it on a grand scale, will mean enduring speeches, mixing ill-matched relatives and friends, and posing for photos in fineries that may never again be worn. But sharing a life together does mark off a radical change in your state and some people do gain from having it publicly acknowledged in a special way.

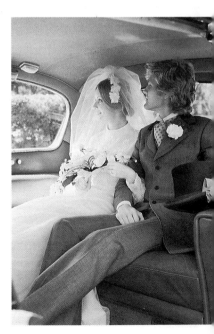

COUPLES NEED TO WEIGH UP FOR THEMSELVES THE PROS AND CONS OF HAVING A TRADITIONAL MARRIAGE.

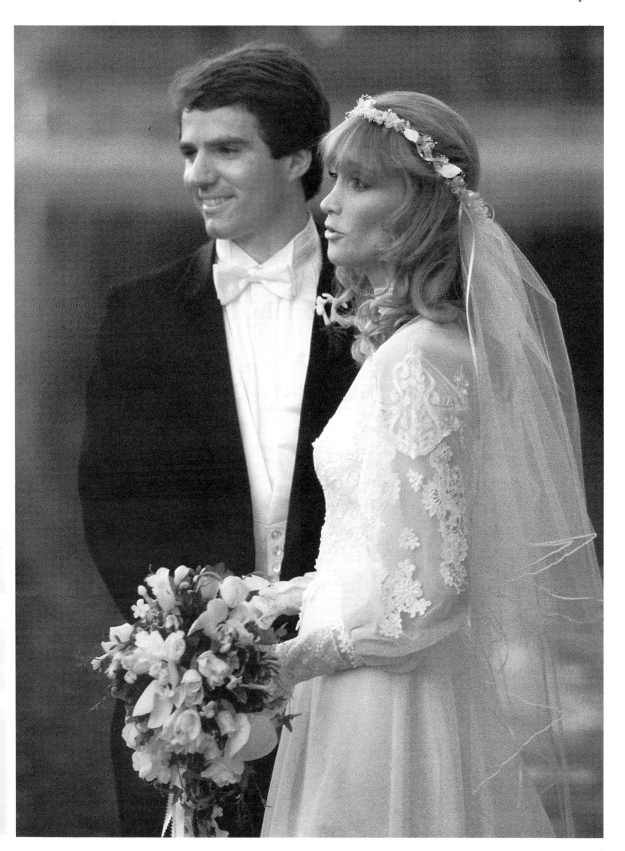

'I want to be free but I need to feel safe'____

Unlike marriage, which has built-in rules about sharing money and possessions, about looking after one another, about being faithful and staying together for a long time, living together tends to be what you want it to be and what you make it. You make the rules. For many, this freedom is what makes cohabitation so attractive. Some people cannot maintain a relationship unless they feel free to walk out at any time, and feeling that they're free to walk out is what keeps them in the relationship.

But this freedom is double-edged. Some people thrive on it, but it makes others feel very insecure, insecure to the point of not being able to make a go of things unless there is some promise of longer-term commitment. The problems begin when one partner starts to make demands which make the other partner feel trapped. There is no better recipe for souring a relationship than one partner feeling tied down and boxed in.

The balance between security and freedom is one we have to juggle with throughout life. We constantly have to weigh up the costs and benefits of being free against those of feeling secure and cocooned, and the break-even point varies with each individual. One person's security will be another's prison. Sometimes couples have quite different ideas about what living together means. One partner may see it as a permanent way of life, the other as a prelude to marriage or as a trial period leading eventually to marriage. The important thing is that you should both be absolutely honest and open with each other about what you expect to give and receive and where you think you're going, and especially when the relationship arouses feelings you don't feel comfortable with.

EVERYDAY CHORES, SUCH AS WORKING OUT THE HOUSEHOLD BILLS OR DOING THE WASHING-UP, ARE NOT THE MOST EXCITING THINGS YOU'LL SHARE, BUT THEY'RE PART OF THE BUSINESS OF LIVING TOGETHER AND NEED NEGOTIATING IF THEY'RE NOT TO CAUSE ROWS.

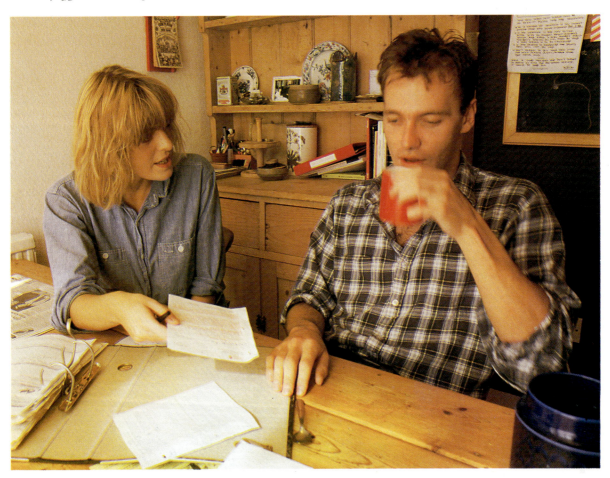

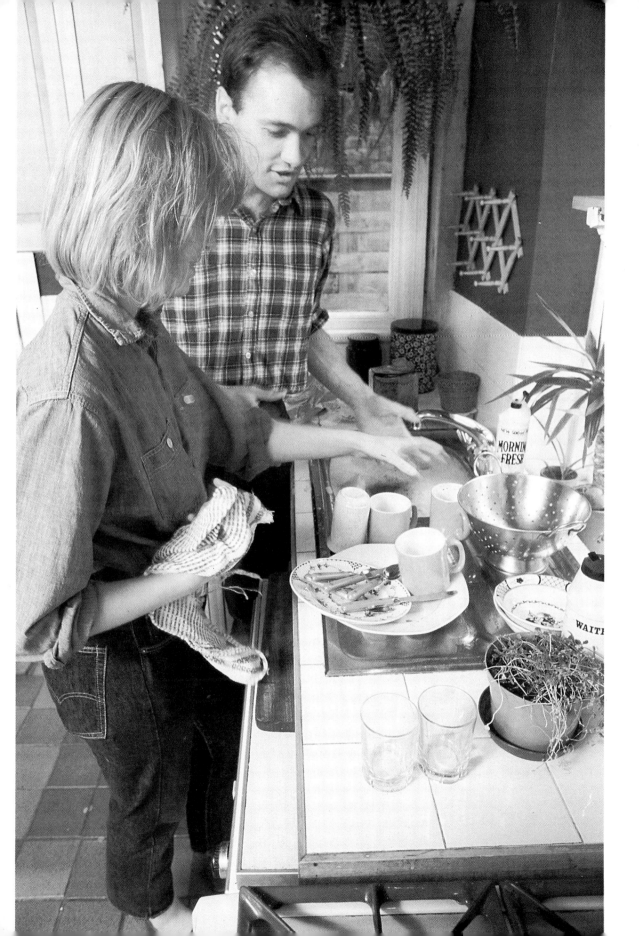

'What about a contract? Is it a good idea?'

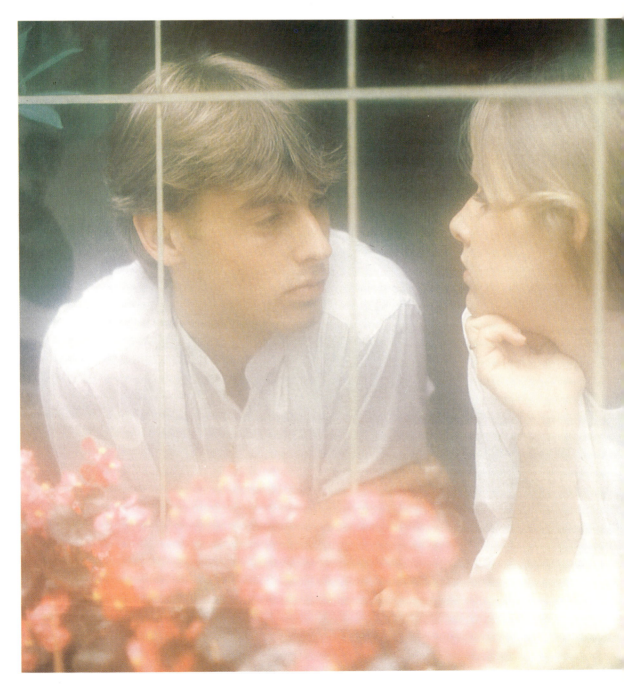

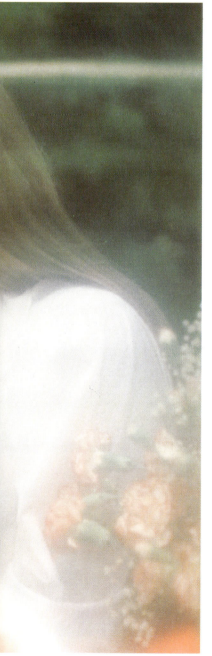

Contracts are as much about rights and freedoms as they are about obligations and restrictions. Because living together does not have the built-in rules that marriage does, some couples feel the need to specify their responsibilities towards each other. Other's don't, saying that love alone is the best guarantee of good behaviour and that the more you have in writing the less you have on trust.

> *'Contracts are all about possessions. They've got nothing to do with how you feel about each other. It's the emotional ties that keep you together, not some legal document.'* BOB

> *'I don't see any need for a contract and I've been living with Mike for three years now. Those people I've seen draw one up, when they've needed it they haven't used it, so it's a complete waste of time.'* SARAH

Of course it may be your reluctance to 'reduce' your relationship to a written document, to a set of obligations enshrined in law, that made you opt for living together rather than marrying in the first place. Besides, when you're seeing life through jointly acquired rose-tinted spectacles the thought of ever needing the safeguards a contract offers is the last thing that goes through your mind.

But there is another side to it. Working out the practical side of the relationship just might reduce the kind of misunderstanding which could sour it. A cohabitation contract can be drawn up specially for the two of you, and it doesn't have to be studded with hereafters, wheretofores and notwithstandings. It can be a simple statement dealing with who owns what and who gets what if you split up, signed by yourselves and two witnesses. Even if it's not legally binding, both of you should regard it as morally binding.

Some couples draw up living-together contracts complete with small print about which chores are carried out by whom and so on. You may feel this is going too far, and certainly very few married couples go to these sort of lengths to avoid potential domestic wrinkles. Yet it is all too easy to start out as you *don't* mean to go on, setting destructive patterns which become hard to break out of. The little things you shrug off during the first flush of romance can become major irritations later. So even if you don't opt for a written contract, try to work out some mutually agreed ground rules *before* you set up home together.

A COHABITATION CONTRACT CAN BE A SIMPLE STATEMENT DEALING WITH WHO OWNS WHAT AND WHO GETS WHAT IF YOU SPLIT UP.

'Meet my POOSSLQ' _____

How do you refer, in public, to the person you live with? Because language takes a while to catch up with social change there are, as yet, no particularly suitable labels. Say 'Meet my husband/neighbour/sister' and everyone knows where they stand. Say 'Meet my mistress/lover' and you feel you're overplaying the sexual side of the relationship. 'Meet my companion/cohabitant' sounds cold and starchy. 'My man' has a 'you Jane, me Tarzan' ring to it, and 'my lady' sounds positively feudal.

Since living together became officially recognized (if not socially approved of) government departments have had to start thinking up suitable titles and tags. In England the Department of Health refers to cohabitants as 'Those Who Are Living Together As Man And Wife' (which shortens to TWALTAMAW) while the US Census Bureau settles for 'Persons Of The Opposite Sex Sharing Living Quarters' (POOSSLQ), which is not exactly the same thing. Saying 'Meet my TWALTAMAW/POOSSLQ' doesn't seem to be catching on.

You have to accept the fact that there will be awkward moments when people introduce you or when you describe your partner. People will refer to him or her by 'um-ing' and 'er-ing' nervously. You can deal with this by being totally honest ('This is Tony who lives with me'), or totally dishonest ('This is Tony, my brother/husband'), or by leaving it to guesswork ('This is Tony').

> *'I usually avoid saying who Gary is. "Boyfriend" sounds twee and doesn't really describe him, "partner" is too formal, and if you come right out with it and say "the man I live with" people might think you're trying to ram the point home to them. Once when we were out , Gary described me as his "fiancée". When I asked him why later, he said he thought it would be less embarrassing for me, but I think he was the embarrassed one.'* DEBBIE

Practically speaking, if you feel comfortable with your description of your partner, other people will feel more at ease. A touch of humour helps. Looking on the positive side, the good thing about there not being a suitable name for people who live together is that you're less likely to be seen as someone else's other half. You're a person in your own right and not an appendage.

PARENTS' ATTITUDES TOWARDS COHABITATION ARE STILL TIED UP WITH THE NOTION THAT SEX OUTSIDE MARRIAGE IS WRONG.

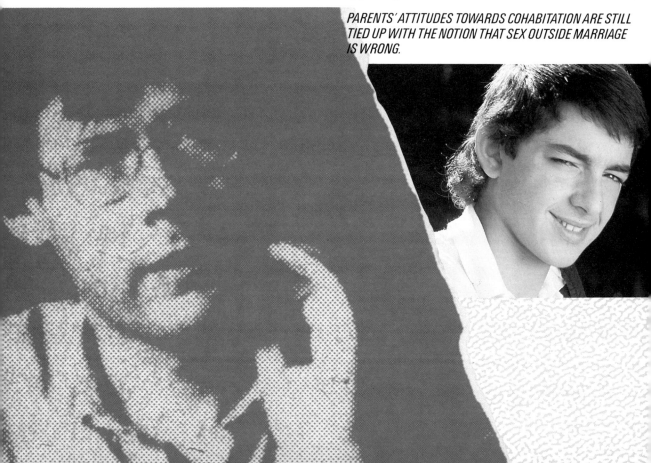

'What will my parents think if we live together?'

Attitudes towards cohabitation are changing dramatically, partly because the practice is now so common. It's difficult to publicly disapprove of something a lot of people are doing. Even Debrett's *Etiquette and Modern Manners*, the top people's guide to impeccable behaviour, now offers advice to live-in lovers and to hostesses perplexed about sleeping arrangements for unmarried couples.

Of course, accepting something done by the populace at large is not the same as accepting something done by our nearest and dearest. Tell your mother that John and Linda are living together and she probably won't turn a hair, but if it's her own kith and kin her attitude may be very different. Sex is the major stumbling block. Attitudes towards cohabitation are still tied up with the notion that sex outside marriage is sinful. The assumption was, and to some extent still is, that the man is having his wicked way with the woman, hence the phrases 'kept woman', 'making a honest woman' of someone by marrying her, and 'living in sin', implying that all cohabitants ever do together is cavort around the bedroom!

'I know a girl who lived with her boyfriend for a couple of years and when she got married her mother came round and gave her a pair of knickers! She must have thought that when she was living with this man she never had her knickers on, but that when she got married she was suddenly going to behave respectably.' ANNA

Parental attitudes are put to their severest test when their cohabiting offspring come to visit them. What should the sleeping arrangements be?

'It's hard for your family to fit in. Mine didn't accept it, my father not for years. No one took me seriously. They didn't like us sleeping together. When we went home they made the beds up in separate rooms and gave us small single ones so that we'd be uncomfortable if we moved over.' JOEL

Some parents find it easier to accept that their son or daughter is living with someone if they feel it is going to lead eventually to marriage. And since parents, almost without exception, place their children's happiness near the top of their list of priorities, their disapproval may fade if they can see you are genuinely happy. Talk things through with them if you can. Explaining why you choose to live as you do is far better than leaving them in the dark, or pretending you are living a life of blameless chastity.

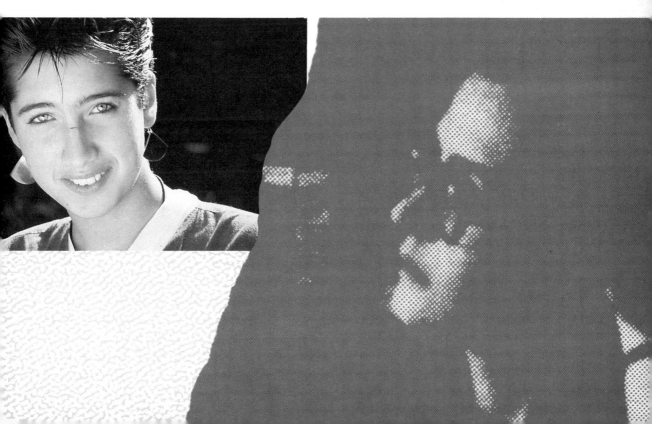

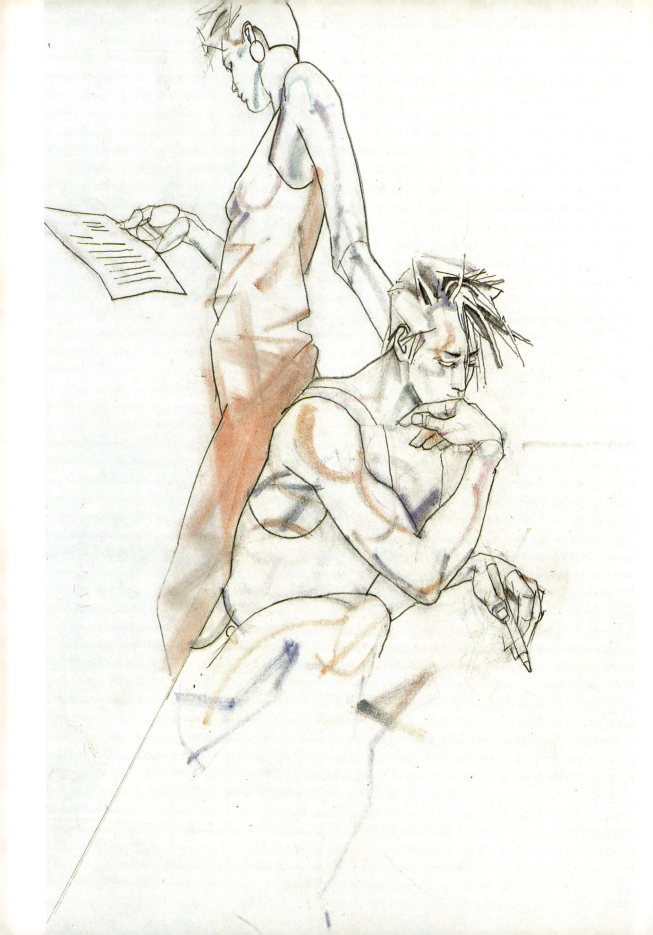

11
Problem Page

Should I show anger?

People show anger in different ways. Some erupt like Mount Vesuvius at the slightest provocation. Others simmer quietly as their temperatures rise, and yet more maintain an icy cold exterior even though everyone knows they're boiling away inside. The instant erupters do have the most obviously disturbing effects on the social calm — on the face of it. But is their approach necessarily the most destructive in the long run?

We tend to receive double messages about anger. Well bred people, we're told, manage to keep their wrath under tight control. Fiery outbursts are not quite the done thing. On the other hand, we hear that to really be self-assertive we need to learn to express anger constructively.

One important point to remember about anger is that it is not an emotion which will easily go away if it's not expressed. Let's look at what might happen in some relationships if anger doesn't find an outlet. Marie, let's say, comes home from the office and is angry that Paul, her student boyfriend, who's been home all day working on his degree, hasn't lifted a finger towards preparing the meal. Marie believes that she has every right to ask Paul for help, but lurking somewhere in her upbringing, she has some old entrenched ideas that men shouldn't be expected to help in the kitchen. They've also had some fairly heated rows before on this topic with disastrous results both for the crockery and for their personal feelings. So though she's actually hopping mad, Marie is afraid of what might happen if she confronts Paul. So she holds her tongue and bottles up her hostility. Until later that is, when little bursts of anger keep bubbling up to the surface, and are expressed as nit-picking niggles which mar the evening. Does he have to leave his papers all over the coffee table/watch this rubbish/smoke another cigarette?

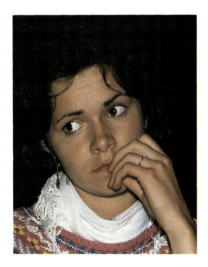

Instead of taking the lid off the pressure cooker, Marie has let the steam phut, phut out of the safety valves around the edge. But Paul is still oblivious to the *real* source of her anger. It just seems to him that she's nagging again. Marie has vented some of her anger, but not in a direct way so that Paul and she could *change* things between them in a positive and permanent way.

Let's look at two other people. Sue and Tom have some niggling sexual problems. Tom would like Sue to take a more active role in sex, to talk whilst they're making love, to be more adventurous maybe, but he can't bring himself to talk to her about it. Instead he withdraws from her, treats her with a sullen reserve, and makes her feel invisible by not looking her in the eye, by interrupting her when she speaks, and by ignoring her presence altogether. The expression of anger here is so subtle that Sue doesn't even know it exists. She just feels that Tom has lost his feelings for her, and so the sexual problem which sparked off his anger gets worse. Sue feels even less inclined to let herself go in lovemaking.

Eventually Tom can't contain his angry feelings any longer, he explodes which makes him feel very guilty and Sue feels shattered. This time, the top has come off the pressure cooker simply as a result of the build-up of steam inside, rather than any control on Tom's part.

Anger can be deflected in numerous other ways. Sometimes if it doesn't find an outlet, it goes inwards, which can be very destructive. Many psychiatrists believe that anger turned inwards is a common cause of depression. Alternately, it may be projected on to another person, who is perhaps easier to deal with — more distant and less emotionally involved, perhaps, than the true focus of angry feelings. But the 'proxy' person won't have a clue why he or she has been singled out for attack. And again, the original source of the anger goes unidentified and therefore unchanged.

Generally speaking, it is better to accept that anger is a normal emotion and to express it as and when it arrives. Don't allow it to get displaced on to another person or situation but tackle its cause directly. Don't store it up, either. That way, when your personal pressure cooker does explode, the effect is so unpleasant that the next time the lid stays on for longer, and so on. Anger *can* be used constructively to convey real feelings of displeasure. Clearing the air now and again allows your more positive feelings to flow freely between you again. So it's OK to blow your top occasionally — but don't make a habit of it.

'We seem to be always getting at each other...'

Those people who claim they never have a quarrel either share the same views on absolutely everything, which must be boring, or else they don't really communicate at all, which must be devastating. If you are close to someone, whether you live with them or not, you both have minds of your own, you must expect that sometimes some things will make you lose your temper.

Sometimes you may find you're quarrelling about pernickety little things which you feel shouldn't really worry you. This may mean that you're harbouring some grudge which is too difficult to talk about. A

common way of handling this is to turn it into a proxy grumble...'You keep on borrowing my comb/cuff links/toothbrush' when actually you mean 'You never talk to me/respond in bed/want my friends to come round.' Money grumbles are often used as a substitute for deeper-rooted grievances. Couples accuse one another of pennypinching, when they're actually protesting about being denied a little tender loving care.

Being aware that these sorts of niggles might be hiding deeper resentments, might help you get to the bottom of real flaws in your relationship. So next time a petty problem crops up, explore it. Why does it bother you so much? If you can do this without blowing a fuse, then there's a chance that a really constructive dialogue might develop. That bone of contention which started you talking might help you prevent chasms opening between you.

ANGER IS A NORMAL EMOTION. BUT DON'T STORE IT UP OR ALLOW IT TO GET DISPLACED ON TO YOUR PARTNER.

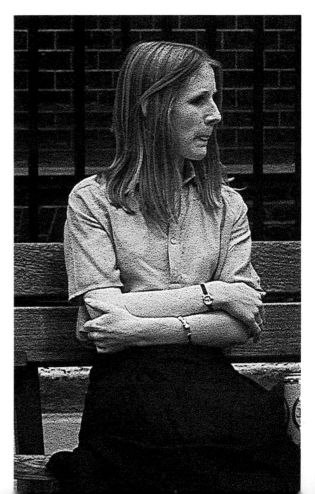

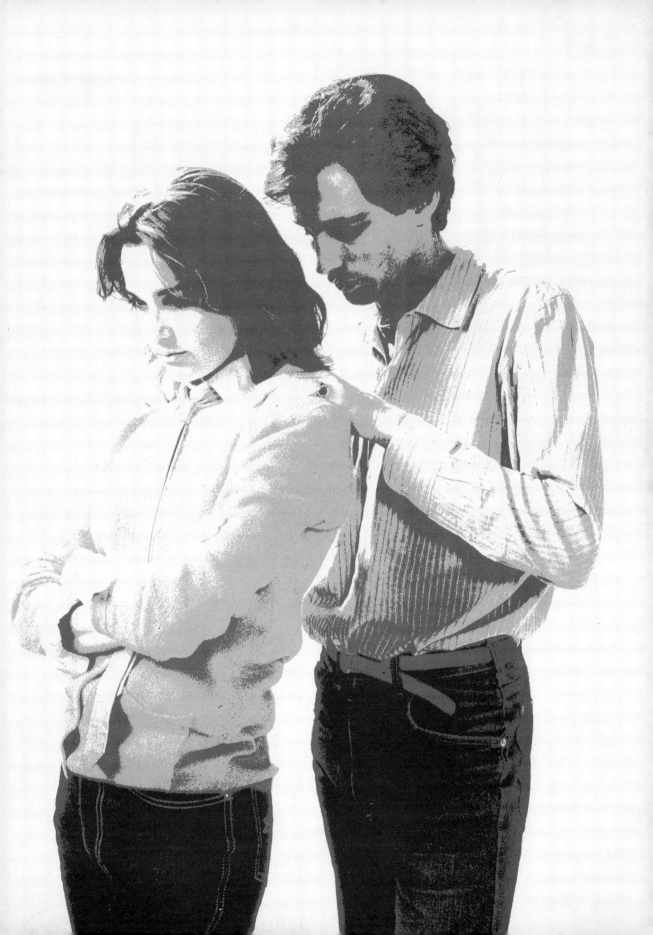

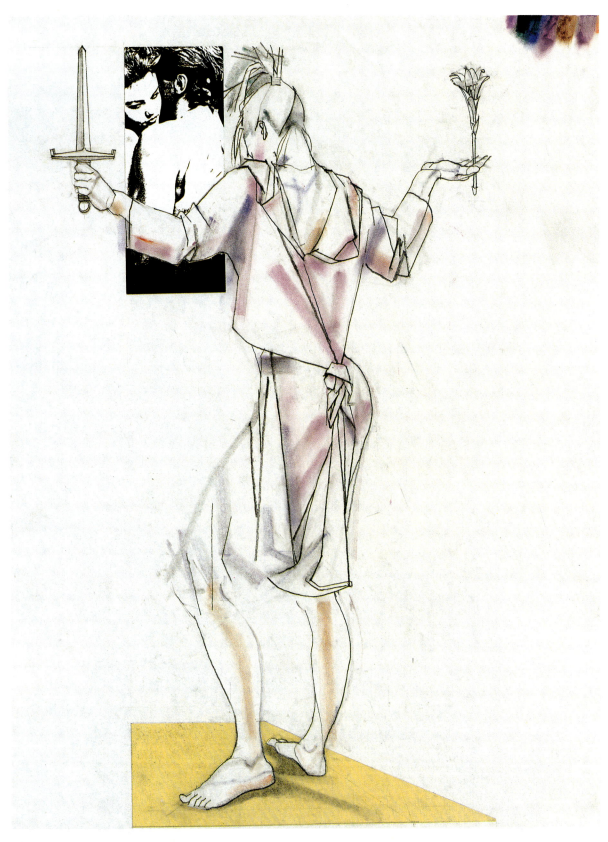

Jealousy

Most of us have been in the grip of the Green Eyed Monster at some time or other; the experience isn't a pleasant one. Although jealousy is triggered by fear of losing someone we love, it can feel far more like hate than love. If we let it get the better of us it can be a very dangerous and destructive force. It was unfounded jealousy that drove Shakespeare's Othello to kill his lovely wife Desdemona. And in France, judges to this day are obliged to show special lenience to people convicted of a murder motivated by jealousy or 'crime passionel'.

The causes of jealousy may be real or imaginary and it's important to be able to tell the difference. Sometimes there are well founded reasons for feeling jealous; perhaps the relationship is a bit shaky or one partner has an incurably roving eye, so that the other understandably feels insecure. But obsessive jealousy, the dark brooding kind that drives people to distraction, is usually built on fantasy and fiction rather than hard facts. If this is the case, it's probably a symptom of deep rooted insecurity and lack of confidence on the part of the possessor. People with a poor sense of their own value will constantly harbour suspicions that their partners are on the look-out for someone better. And they'll go to any lengths to have their suspicions confirmed — sifting through coat pockets, listening in on 'phone calls and generally playing super spy. It's not so much that they love someone else too much, as that they don't love themselves enough.

The irony is that this sort of obsessive jealousy can provoke just the sort of behaviour the jealous person most fears, as this experience shows:

'I've been living with my boyfriend for just over a year now and although we get on quite well generally, his fits of jealousy are really getting me down. When we go to parties or have drinks with friends, he watches me like a hawk and listens to my conversations with other men even if he's talking to someone else. When we get back we have terrible rows and he accuses me of flirting and making up to other men. Just recently I've taken to sticking to the women to talk to, but what I really feel like doing is having a fling just to show him.' CLAIRE

Claire obviously feels she might as well be hanged for a sheep as a lamb. 'I've-had-the-punishment, let's-see-what-the-crime-feels-like' sort of logic. Eventually the partner is driven to be unfaithful and the jealousy is self-fulfilling.

What can we do about it? We can't stop feeling jealous. The emotion is much too powerful for us to have that sort of control. What matters is how we reflect on it and how much we learn about ourselves as a result. Getting to the bottom of the reasons for feeling this way is an important start. Are you feeling insecure and blaming your partner? Is this jealousy a feature of all your relationships or a one off? Is your partner just inheriting some old grievances? Is there enough trust between you? Are you off-loading your own secret guilty yearnings for sexual freedom onto your partner? Talking things over will help get things in perspective. Causing a scene will not. Jealous rages may push an innocent partner into the crime they're accused of, and give guilty ones the excuse they've been looking for.

But if there is a deep seated problem of insecurity then the chances are that the problem will turn up again in a later relationship, and you may need to get some specialist advice to help you deal with it.

If you're on the receiving end of jealousy, try to find ways of showing your loyalty. This doesn't mean treating people any other way than comes naturally to you. But it might mean showing that mildly flirtatious behaviour doesn't threaten your relationship in any way. A close friend can go a long way towards building feelings of trust and security which were maybe missing in an important earlier relationship.

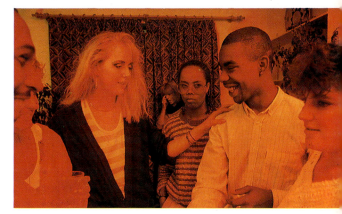

Guilt

Guilt is the emotion we may feel when we please ourselves at someone else's expense. In a civilised society there have to be rules and regulations to safeguard people's interests and to ensure that everyone gets a fair deal. We feel guilt when we flout them and get on selfishly with our own thing. It's our internal voice of conscience punishing us for being selfishly indulgent.

If we do something hurtful to another person then we would expect to feel some guilt. But some people often carry tremendously burdensome packages of guilt around, quite out of proportion to their actual crime. Wallowing in guilt about deeds long gone or fairly trivial is not at all constructive. So if you feel someone else is forcing a hefty ball and chain on you, you have to think carefully about whether you've earned it.

Having clearly thought out ideas about what is right and wrong doesn't just mean taking on board other people's moral codes unthinkingly. The central question in your own personal blueprint/code is 'How can I make sure that what I do causes as little hurt to as few people as possible?' It's impossible to please everyone all the time. We'll never reach the point where some of our needs don't conflict with someone else's. Those who completely ignore their own needs are either martyrs or masochists and neither are very easy to live with. If you give in to guilt unquestioningly, you'll probably be behaving so virtuously that eventually someone else starts to feel guilty.

So accept your share of blame, by all means, when you've done something to deserve it. But if a friend is making you feel constantly guilty, ask yourself whether they have the right to burden you so. If you're accused of being too friendly to other people, for example, ask yourself whether this might not be because the person making the accusation feels ill at ease with people, and that their comparison with your gregarious self is perhaps too cruel. Guilt should never be inflicted on a friend as a weapon to make them toe a line you didn't agree to in the first place.

Depression

Everyone feels fed up from time to time. There are doldrum days when nothing seems to go right, when everything seems a real effort. We feel worthless and inadequate; self-esteem is low and anxiety levels are high. Everyday life seems both pointless and meaningless. In fact the symptoms of being generally down in the dumps are very like those of real depression. So how do you tell the difference?

Psychologists make the distinction between the type of depression which is linked clearly to a particularly distressing event or troublesome period of life, and the kind which has no apparent cause. The first type is often a reaction to loss — the breakup of a relationship or the loss of a job, for example. And it's often associated with important but stressful transitions in life — leaving college or getting married, perhaps.

Depression may also have a physical cause; it may be hormonal, for example. Women often suffer from bouts of depression before a period or after the birth of a baby. In both sexes it can be related to fatigue, when the body's defences are low.

More worrying is the kind of depression which doesn't seem to observe any of the rules of reason. It doesn't seem to be connected with anything you can put your finger on that's wrong (though nothing seems very right). It stops you getting on with your life and with the people in it, and it stops you being effective; it saps energy and denies you pleasure or satisfaction in anything.

> *I didn't feel like doing anything. Everything I touched seemed to turn to stone. It didn't matter how hard I tried, I just couldn't do anything right. I had absolutely no faith in myself. I would go through agonies about giving in a piece of work at college. In the end I couldn't even get myself there. I stayed in bed. I wasn't coping with anything and I felt I'd reached breaking point.*
> HELEN

Whatever the underlying reason for it, what is clear is that it is *not* normal to be emotionally out of sorts *all* the time. This kind of unfocused depression is more properly called an illness than a mood, but it's not an illness which will earn its victim anything like as much sympathy as a bout of 'flu or a boil. Yet it's important to remember that the pain and despair of depression *can* be fatal — as many coroner's verdicts in suicide cases have shown. It is also very real to the sufferer, and he or she can't just snap out of it.

> *People told me to grow up and accept responsibility, think of others worse off than myself, or plunge myself into some absorbing interest. But none of this makes any sense when you're depressed. You're not interested in anything outside of yourself, you're completely wrapped up in your own problems. Friends can remind you of how lucky you are, of how much*

you've got going for you and so on, but you just can't see it. When you're depressed, all your thoughts are negative, just black. TERRY

So what *can* you do about depression? A visit to your GP might be helpful, but since doctors don't always have the time to get to the bottom of the problem, they do tend to reach for their prescription pads. Anti-depressant pills may give temporary relief but medicine isn't the best way to change moods. It certainly isn't the solution in all situations. There's a natural link between sadness and depression and if something deeply depressing happens — the loss of a loved one, for example — banishing the feelings with drugs won't help. The depression will often surface again when the treatment stops.

There are some things that you can do to keep depressive moods at bay. Keeping a diary might help identify what triggers depression in you personally. It might be late nights, overwork, being alone too much. Do your best to arrange things so that such events don't coincide. If you know there are stressful times ahead in one sphere of life, try to cut down or control the stress level in another.

If self-esteem (or lack of it) is a real problem for you, use your friends to help build it up. See the ones who do this most effectively, and give those who put you down a miss. When we're feeling bad about ourselves, it takes an enormous amount of courage to face up to friends at all. But talking through problems both when you're up *and* when you're down will help you put things in perspective.

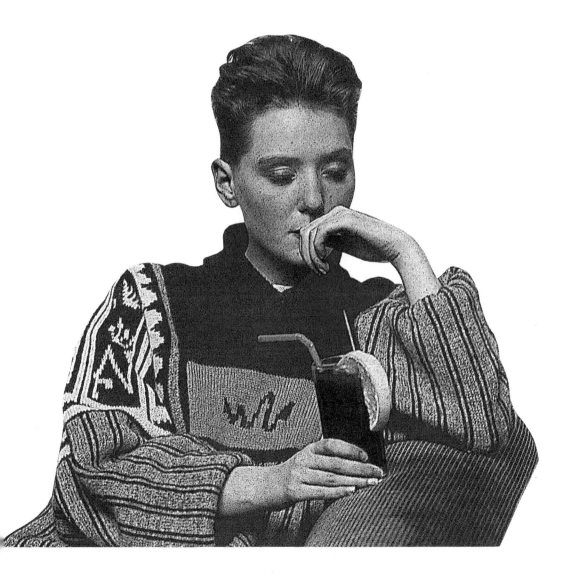

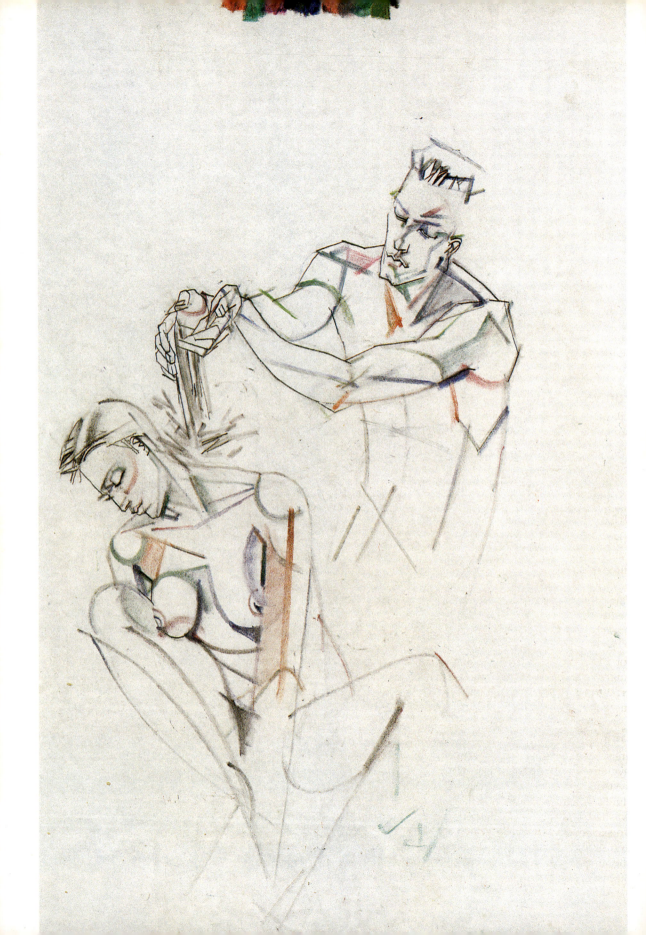

12
Health matters

In this chapter you will find basic information on some of the commonest ailments which can affect the male and female genital and reproductive organs. Some are simply infections which find the primary and secondary sex organs particularly hospitable! Not all of them are spread by sexual contact.

Forewarned is forearmed

Like any other part of the body, our sex organs need daily care and attention. We don't think twice about cleaning our teeth after a meal and paying regular visits to the dentist, but we tend to neglect our genital area, perhaps because it's tucked away out of sight. But like any other part of the body, our sex organs need daily care and attention — maybe more so because the genital area is particularly prone to infection. The delicate membranes are easily torn and bruised, allowing germs to get in.

Several germs which choose the genital area as their home produce irritation, mild inflammation and discharge. Apart from their nuisance value, these may not seem very serious in themselves, but they can have dire side-effects. Symptoms which may seem bothersome in the short term if they hinder lovemaking have the potential, in the long term, to cause sterility and leave you unable to have children. So don't ignore or neglect any discharge or irritation, however slight. It may clear up on its own, but by that time the damage may have been done.

Some infections don't produce noticeable symptoms in everyone, but for all that they may be wreaking havoc undercover. So if you think you might be at risk, if you're going through a phase when your love life is a bit erratic and you're changing partners, go to your doctor for a check-up — just as you'd go to the dentist.

Genital hygiene

Treat your genitals with respect, and pay particular attention to personal hygiene. To some extent our bodies have their own built-in cleaning systems. In women, a healthy vagina, for example, naturally produces fluids which flush it out and lubricate it. These should *not* be douched or washed out. When a cat licks herself clean, she doesn't wash off the saliva! The slightly earthy smell of these secretions has a powerful erotic appeal, and shouldn't be deodorized out of existence. Only when the fluids reach the air and are allowed to become stale will they harbour germs and offensive smells, so washing the outer genital folds is essential. In men, a

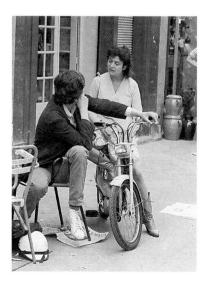

white waxy secretion called smegma is produced under the foreskin of an uncircumcised penis. If it is not regularly washed away, it too develops an unpleasant smell and can be a breeding ground for germs.

Simple hygiene measures like washing your sex organs and anus every day, wiping your bottom from front to back (to avoid spreading germs from the anus), keeping caps and diaphragms clean, checking you haven't left a tampon in place, are all that is needed. Keep an eye open for signs of trouble and use the pages that follow to help you identify them. Think of hygiene and vigilance as body maintenance rather than repair . A few minutes prevention is better than weeks or months off the road!

Prevention is better than cure

Sexually transmitted diseases are on the increase. Many people blame permissiveness and a drop in moral standards, and it is true that freer lifestyles and an increased amount of travelling have raised the risk of infection, but ignorance and prejudice also keep the figures high. If people think they've caught something shameful and degrading they tend to keep quiet about it rather than seek medical advice. Yet if everyone who suspected they had a sexually transmitted disease went to a clinic for treatment, and if their partners did too, then the diseases could be stamped out rapidly.

If you suspect you have any of the diseases described in this chapter, you should get medical treatment straight away. Even if you have no symptoms, but know you have been taking risks, go for regular checkups. You can count yourself as courting above average risks if you have more than one sexual partner, or if your partner makes love to one or more people besides you. You're a high risk candidate if you have several partners each of whom in turn has several partners. Here are some sensible precautions you can take.

■ **Do be choosy about who you have sex with.**

■ **Don't have sex with a second person too soon after the first.** Diseases can be passed on immediately after they are contracted, although the symptoms may not appear straight away.

■ **Do be fastidious about personal hygiene.** Genital folds and wrinkles make excellent homes for bugs — they are warm, moist and cosy. This doesn't mean using commercial preparations to keep fresh — they can often do more harm than good by irritating the skin and providing tiny cuts for the germs to enter. But it does mean being scrupulously clean about daily washing.

■ **Don't ignore an unusual discharge or a change of colour in your usual discharge.** If the discharge stains your briefs more than usual, causes itching or discomfort, or has an unpleasant smell, regard it as suspect. The chances are that it's a mild infection that can be easily cured, but only a doctor can tell you that for sure.

■ **Don't take it for granted that you are infection-free if early symptoms disappear.** This may be the case — things do clear up on their own — but symptoms of some diseases can put in an initial appearance and then go into hiding. You may still be infectious and the infection could lead to further complications.

■ **Do tell your partner about any unusual symptoms.** This may be embarrassing, but he or she needs to know if they've passed an infection to you, or if they can catch it from you. Sheaths only lessen the risk of infection, they do not eliminate it. So if you know you've got a sexually transmitted infection you should abstain completely until your doctor says you are in the clear.

■ **Don't kid yourself that dirty towels or toilet seats are the culprits.** Scientists who've tried to grow bugs on toilet seats have had poor success rates! And even if you didn't *catch* an infection through sexual contact, you can still *pass it on* by this means.

■ **Do seek medical advice.** You can find the name of your nearest clinic from your doctor, from your local hospital, from your telephone directory or from some of the organizations listed at the end of the book. Few clinics today still have the formidable name of 'venereal disease clinics'; they're more likely to be found under Department of Genito-Urinary Medicine, STD Clinic or Department of Genital Medicine.

■ **Don't make love if you have any reason to believe that you have an infection. Wait until you have had it cured.**

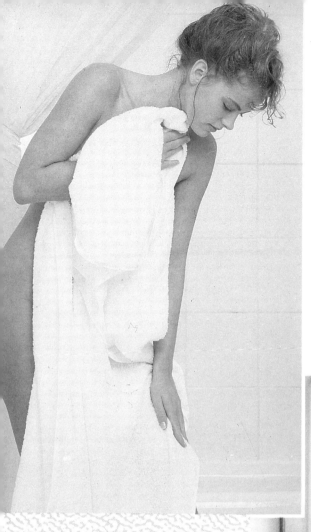

PERSONAL HYGIENE IS AN IMPORTANT PART OF A
PREVENTIVE HEALTH CARE STRATEGY.

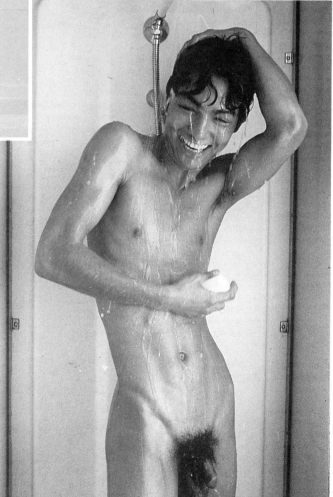

'What happens when I go to a clinic?'

Some STD clinics are organized on a walk-in basis, others on an appointment system. Checking beforehand will save a wait. If you turn up as a new patient, you're booked in and asked to give name, address and date of birth, together with some brief details of your previous medical history. You'll also be asked what brought you there, whether you have any symptoms and what they are, whether you've been in contact with a person you know to be infected, and other relevant information, such as when you last had sex, whether you have any drug allergies and so on. You will not be asked to divulge information about who you had sex with, and the staff will treat any information you give them in complete confidence (even, in some clinics, to the point of giving you a number so that other patients can't identify you). Only if you have an infection will you be advised to tell those you might have passed it on to, and if it does turn out to be a serious infection — like gonorrhoea — then a little more pressure will be put on you to do this.

'What will they do to me?'

After the initial interview, you can expect a thorough examination. Whatever their symptoms, everyone is given a routine blood test for syphilis, and you may be asked to give a urine sample. Swabs are taken from the penis and the vagina, and if you've told the clinic you've had oral or anal sex, swabs will be taken from the throat and back passage too. Some organisms, such as pubic lice, can be detected simply by taking a look at the sex organs, so you can expect the doctor to carry out a fairly thorough genital search. Some results will be available on the day, others go off to the lab and may take a few days, but you'll be informed as soon as they come through.

FREER LIFESTYLES HAVE BEEN PARTLY RESPONSIBLE FOR THE SPREAD OF SEXUALLY TRANSMITTED DISEASES — BUT FEAR AND PREJUDICE KEEP THE FIGURES HIGH TOO.

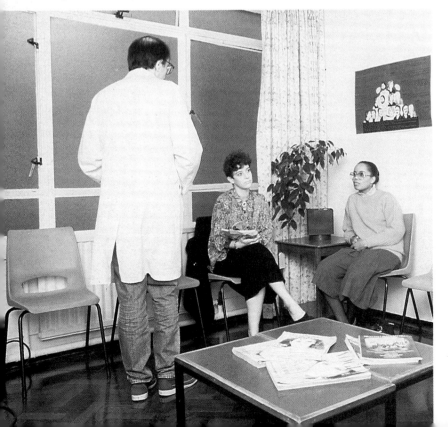

SEXUALLY TRANSMITTED DISEASE CLINICS ARE NOT THE UNFRIENDLY PLACES THEY ONCE WERE — TODAY'S WALK-IN CLINICS ARE WARM, DISCREET AND CHEERFUL.

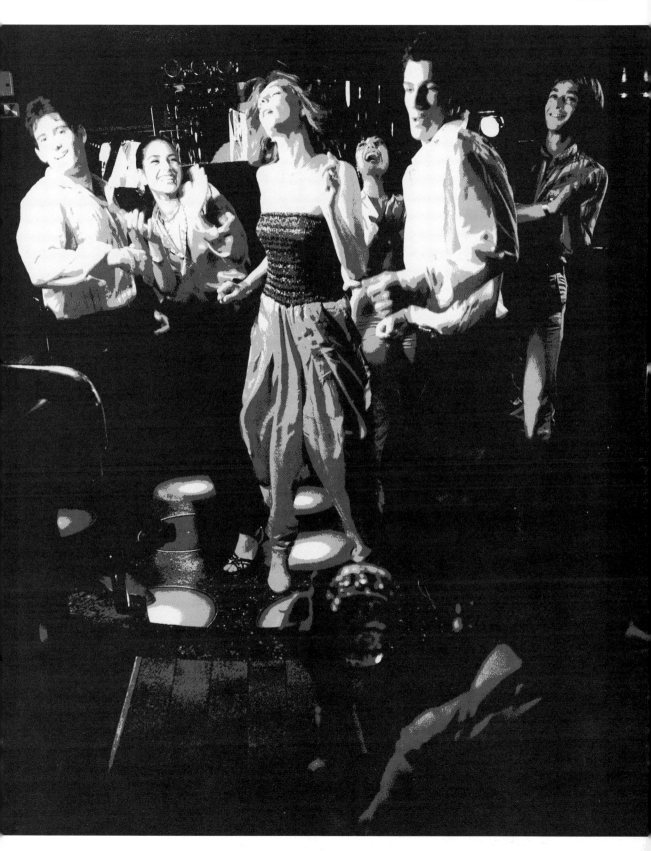

Sexually transmitted diseases

GONORRHOEA

Sometimes called the 'clap', 'drip' or 'dose', gonorrhoea has been around for hundreds of years, probably since Biblical times. The bacteria responsible for the disease are shaped like kidney beans and can only be seen through a microscope. They survive only in the warmth and moisture of the body and are passed on only during genital, oral or anal contact.

Symptoms   The incubation period is three to seven days, so symptoms would appear within a week. For centuries, people thought the disease only affected males, because females often show no symptoms at all. Nine out of ten men with the disease have obvious symptoms, while six out of ten women don't notice a thing. This is one reason why gonorrhoea has been hard to control. A woman will often seek treatment only if she knows her partner is infected.

Men

● Pain when passing urine

● Yellow discharge from the penis

● Infection of anus sometimes causes discharge and irritation

Women

● Burning feeling when passing urine

● Unusual vaginal discharge

● (Occasionally) symptoms of fever, chill, pain in the abdomen and joints.

● Infection of anus sometimes causes discharge and irritation

Treatment   Unchecked, gonorrhoea can cause inflammation of the genital area or, more rarely, the prostate gland in men, and can lead to a permanent inability to have children in women. More rarely, the bacteria can spread through the body to the heart, liver, skin or joints. A course of penicillin is the most effective cure, except where the sufferer is allergic to the drug, when other antibiotics can be used. Some 'superbugs' have evolved recently with a built-in resistance to penicillin, but as yet this is not a major problem. No cure protects against a repeat bout of infection; having gonorrhoea once provides no immunity to a second attack.

SYPHILIS

This disease takes its name from the Greek shepherd Syphilis who angered Apollo by cursing him and ceasing to worship him, and was smitten with the disease as a punishment. The idea of syphilis as the 'wages of sin' has never been completely abandoned. The disease has always been steeped in dread, fear and mystery, perhaps because of its horrific complications. Yet today it is relatively rare and easy to cure. It affects men more than women (the ratio is about three to one) and gay men more than straight men. First symptoms appear anything between nine and ninety days after infection.

Symptoms   These are the same for men and women. Untreated, the disease passes through several different stages, producing different symptoms at each stage.

● **Stage 1.** Primary. A red bump about the size of a pea and called a chancre (pronounced 'shanker') appears on the genital area or more rarely the lip, tongue or anus, at the point where the germ invaded. This painless lump opens up into a red sore but does not bleed.

● **Stage 2:** Secondary. A non-irritating rash turning brownish in colour appears all over the body. 'Flu-like symptoms, run-down feeling, mouth sores, and occasional hair loss.

● **Stage 3:** No symptoms. The germ appears to have retreated but in fact is attacking every organ in the body.

● **Late Stage.** Damage to heart and central nervous system, leading to paralysis, blindness, deafness, madness and eventually death.

Treatment   Nowadays, the chances of a case of syphilis being allowed to get beyond the early stages to the deadly later stages are extremely remote. In the first and second stages, syphilis is easily cured by penicillin, and even the third stage will respond to the drug, though it takes considerably longer.

HERPES

Very few people had heard of herpes before its burst of publicity in recent years. Although it is thought of as a 'new' form of STD, it was known to the ancient Greeks. Herpes affects only three out of every hundred people going for treatment in STD clinics and, although it is an irritating condition, most people learn to live with it — it doesn't wreck their love lives or their sanity.

The disease comes in two forms, herpes Type 1 and

herpes Type 2, sometimes described as attacking above and below the belt respectively. Herpes Type 1 attacks the upper body, usually the area around the mouth and nose, whereas herpes Type 2 attacks the genital and anal area.

The virus produces something like a cold sore which can be passed on during oral sex, during intercourse, or transferred on a finger from mouth to genitals. After an attack, the herpes virus goes to ground in the bundle of nerve cells at the base of the spine. It manages to cause a repeat attack perhaps two or three times a year, and this is often triggered by stress or being run down. Some people who get a first attack, though, never get another one and most of those who *do* find the later outbreaks are milder, heal faster, are not so painful, and are less likely to produce the feverishness which accompanied the first attack.

Because of all the herpes panic recently, sufferers get the feeling they have to give up sex for life. This is not so. It's OK to have sex between attacks as long as there are no active sores or blisters, and as long as there are no signs of an attack coming on.

Symptoms These are similar in both men and women.

● (Particularly in the first attack) an unwell feeling, swollen glands, headaches and feverishness

● Tenderness, tingling or itching around the area where a sore is going to break out

● Clusters or blisters on the penis, vulva or vagina which break to form painful open sores which later crust over

● Pain when passing urine

Treatment Although there is no real cure for herpes as yet, the disease often clears up on its own within a few years. A preparation called Acyclovir, which can be obtained on prescription, has helped many people control their symptoms. Anything which lessens the pain is worth a try. Warm baths help and if passing urine is painful, do it in the bath. Salt added to the water is often soothing. Witch hazel or surgical spirit (from chemists) helps to dry out the sores. Avoid anything which rubs the skin, and leave the sores open to the air whenever possible. Always wash your hands with soap and water after touching sores.

AIDS (Acquired Immune Deficiency Syndrome)
AIDS was not officially classified as an STD until the summer of 1981. Since then, the disease has spread and become front page news throughout the United States and Europe, as no victim diagnosed as having AIDS for two or more years has so far survived. Media attention has greatly exaggerated the incidence of AIDS though the severity of the disease can't be over-estimated. French and American researchers believe they have now identified the virus that causes it.

The disease is thought to be spread through body fluids such as blood and semen, so haemophiliacs and intravenous drug users are high risk groups. The other group most at risk is the homosexual community. The immune system of a body attacked by the AIDS virus breaks down, the body loses its ability to fight invading organisms that cause disease, and pneumonia, cancer and other serious diseases then take hold.

Symptoms These are the same for men and women.

● Low-grade, persistent fever

● A dry cough that is not a result of smoking or a cold

● Shortness of breath

● Unaccountable loss of weight

● Fatigue and blurred vision

● Persistent and severe headaches

● Swollen glands in neck and under arms

● Creamy-white patches on tongue

● Persistent itching around anus

● Persistent diarrhoea or stomach upsets

● Cuts and infections that do not heal as quickly as they should

● Persistent skin rashes and discolorations

Obviously many of these symptoms also occur with other diseases or complaints. Only if many of the symptoms occur at the same time and you are at high risk should you consult your doctor, and even then you are extremely unlikely to have AIDS.

GENITAL WARTS
Once regarded as a minor medical problem, genital warts are beginning to be taken far more seriously now that evidence is building up that they might play a part in the development of cancer of the cervix in women. They look like common skin warts but seem much larger when they're clustered together, and are spread by genital or anal contact, or from the fingers to the anus. In men they're found mainly on the penis, in women in the vagina, and in gay men around the anus.

Symptoms Apply to both men and women:

● In moist areas: painless cauliflower-like growths, reddish pink in colour, varying in size from a pinhead to a grape

● On dry skin: smaller, harder and yellowish grey in colour

Treatment As yet there is no simple, safe and effective treatment which can be carried out at home. Medical techniques include freezing warts off with liquid nitrogen, burning them by a process called cauterization or, if they are large enough, cutting them out. There are lotions which get rid of warts for some people, but they tend to harm the surrounding skin unless they are washed off after a few hours.

PUBIC LICE (Crabs)
The crab-like appearance of these unsavoury creatures earns them their slang name. They are blood-sucking wingless insects about the size of a pinhead which inhabit the genital area, clinging onto pubic and other hairs with their hind legs. Infestations pass from one person to another, normally through sexual contact, but also from shared towels, bedding or clothes. Pubic lice multiply rapidly; the female lays about eight eggs (nits) a day which stick to the hair roots and hatch in about seven days.

Symptoms These are the same in both men and women.

● Itching around the genital area

● The lice can be seen moving about

● Inflammation and infection sometimes follows the bites

Treatment One way of getting rid of crabs is to shave off the hair in the pubic region, but a brand new razor must be used, and then discarded, and care must be taken not to nick the skin. Conventional treatment is by applying lotions, ointments and shampoos containing lice-killing chemicals. These can be bought over the counter in chemists, or obtained from a clinic.

SCABIES
Scabies is caused by tiny mites which burrow under the skin causing small wavy lines to appear with a minute blister at one end containing the mite. They are spread by direct sexual contact or by dirty clothes which contain the mites or their eggs. Symptoms develop about a month after mites infest the body.

Symptoms These are the same in men and women.

● Tiny black or white lines under the skin, chiefly on the webs of the fingers, the wrists, elbows, armpits, breasts and buttocks, though rarely the genitals

● Inflammation and often unbearable itching around the burrows

Treatment Fresh clean clothing and regular baths are essential to prevent reinfection. Special preparations in lotion form are applied to the whole body from the neck down.

Genital Infections
Several germs which live in the genital area produce symptoms of discharge, itching, soreness and inflammation of the penis, vagina or anus. Often these are a result of sexual contact, but many can just as easily be due to taking the pill, being run down, not paying enough attention to personal hygiene, or borrowing infected towels or clothing. Some of the commonest germs are listed below with their symptoms and methods of treatment.

There are simple precautionary measures you can take to prevent and control all of them:

■ Wear cotton rather than nylon pants.

■ Baggy jeans are better than tightly fitting ones.

■ Don't use perfumed toilet preparations.

■ Avoid intercourse if there is any broken or tender skin in the area around the genitals.

THRUSH (candidiasis, candidosis or moniliasis)
Thrush, an irritating condition affecting mainly women, is caused by a yeast or fungus (*Candida*) which flourishes in damp, dark and airless nooks and crannies. Normally it lurks in the vaginal area and is prevented from doing any harm by the acid environment of the vagina and by natural bacteria present in the body. Anything which disturbs these conditions will quickly encourage the yeast to grow. Taking the pill can do it, and so can antibiotics, because they destroy *Candida*'s natural enemies. The infection can be, but is not always, spread by sexual contact. Borrowed towels, swimwear and underwear can also transfer it.

Symptoms These affect mainly women, as mentioned above, but are similar in men.

● Irritation can range from slight discomfort and itching to intense soreness, burning and ulceration

● White patches resembling cottage cheese appear on inflamed areas, which may bleed when dislodged

● Intercourse may be painful

● A watery to thickish yellow discharge is often present. This has the characteristic, and not unpleasant, smell of new mown hay or freshly baked bread

● In men, the yeast can cause irritation under the foreskin of the penis

Treatment Thrush can be resistant to treatment. Antifungal preparations do the trick for most women; these come in the form of suppositories (small, waxy, torpedo-shaped tablets which you slip into the vagina) or special creams which can be applied to other areas. The most stubborn cases have been known to respond to live goat's milk yogurt inserted into the vagina by smearing it liberally onto a tampon. Absolute cleanliness is essential and the genital area should be kept clean, cool and dry. Tight fitting jeans and briefs, and all man-made fibres make the condition worse and should be replaced by looser fitting and preferably cotton, clothes. Tights should have an open gusset. (These can be bought ready-made, otherwise cut a hole in existing ones.)

NSU (Non-Specific Urethritis), **NGU** (Non-Gonococcal Urethritis) or **PGU** (Post-Gonococcal Urethritis)
This infection accounts for by far the largest number of cases treated in STD clinics. It is called 'urethritis' because it causes inflammation of the urethra (the tube in both men and women that conveys urine from the bladder to the outside), and 'non-specific' because laboratory tests usually rule out gonorrhoea but cannot pinpoint the exact cause of the infection. *Chlamydia* (see below) is thought to be the culprit in at least 60 per cent of cases; but in many others there is no link with sexual contact. Men whose partners are free from infection and who only have sex with that partner can still become infected. NSU has an incubation period of seven to fourteen days.

Symptoms

● Pain when passing urine

● Discharge from bladder opening (women)

● Discharge from the penis

Treatment Both partners need to go on a course of antibiotics, and must abstain from sexual contact until the condition has cleared up — tests will show when this has happened. NSU can be difficult to cure.

TRICHOMONIASIS ('Trich')
This is a very common condition affecting as many as one in five women at some time during their lives, but less common in men. The organism responsible lurks in the folds of the vulva or under the foreskin of the penis, causing irritation and soreness. Infection can be spread by sexual contact or by shared towels or splashes on toilet seats. Symptoms show up seven to twenty-eight days after infection.

Symptoms Many of those infected show no symptoms, or only one of the following:

● Foul-smelling greenish discharge

● Pain during intercourse

● Irritation and redness of vulva

● An outbreak of cystitis (see later) in women

● Irritation, soreness and redness of the penis in men

Treatment Several drugs taken by mouth will kill off the 'trich' germ — brand names include oral Flagyl and Naxogin.

GARDNERELLA
A vaginal inflammation caused by bacteria.

Symptoms

● Heavy and unusual discharge with an unpleasant fishy smell, greyish and possibly frothy

● Sometimes irritation

Treatment Pills called Flagyl, or Ampicillin, are taken by mouth and sometimes combined with the use of sulfa creams or suppositories.

CHLAMYDIA (see also NSU and PID)
Chlamydia organisms are a cross between bacteria and viruses. They cause a variety of infections, some of which are sexually transmitted and affect the sex organs of both men and women. If left untreated, they can cause NSU in men and far more serious, pelvic inflammatory disease or PID (see later) in women, possibly leading to infertility, so prompt attention is essential. IUD users need to be especially vigilant.

Symptoms

● A variable amount of vaginal discharge and occasionally some bleeding in women

● Discharge from the penis in men

● Occasional irritation and itching

● If *Chlamydia* leads to more widespread infection, any of the symptoms listed under PID may be present.

Treatment Detected early, chlamydial infections can quickly be cleared up with antibiotics — like tetracycline — taken by mouth.

PID (Pelvic Inflammatory Disease)

This is the name given to infections which have spread beyond the genital area to the reproductive organs of women. Inflammation and infection do not restrict themselves to the pelvis (the basin-shaped structure formed by the bones in the lower abdomen) but spreads to the womb, the tubes along which the eggs pass, and the ovaries.

Infections can cause the tubes to be blocked so that neither eggs nor sperm can pass along them. They can also lead to scarring of the delicate membranes of the reproductive tract. All this adds up to some women having difficulty becoming pregnant. The idea of having children may seem to belong to the distant future, but if you avoid problems now, you could avoid a cause of infertility later.

Symptoms

● Pain in the abdomen or lower back

● Fever, ill health and tiredness

● Vaginal discharge

● Heavy or irregular periods

● Nausea or sickness

Treatment   PID can be successfully treated with antibiotics, either taken orally in the early stages, or intravenously in later stages. Sometimes surgical removal of the infected organs may be necessary.

CYSTITIS

Cystitis is an inflammation of the lining of the bladder and the urethra (the tube leading from the bladder to the outside of the body). It is extremely common, affecting something like half of all women at some time in their lives, and excruciatingly painful. Infection is usually the cause, because the bladder opening, bowel opening and vaginal opening are close enough together in women for germs to pass easily from one to the other. But the complaint can also be due to bruising of the bladder opening by an over-enthusiastic penis, hence the name 'honeymoon cystitis'.

Symptoms

● A feeling of wanting to pass urine constantly, even though there is little to pass

● A burning or scalding feeling on passing urine

● Blood and maybe pus in the urine

● Pain low down in the abdomen and back

Treatment If there are signs of infection, cystitis can be treated by relieving the symptoms. The quickest and most effective way of doing this is to flush as much liquid through the body as possible. Drink half a pint of water at 20-minute intervals. A teaspoonful of bicarbonate of soda dissolved in the water will help to make the urine less acid and stop it burning; potassium citrate (in tablet or liquid form) is even better if you can get someone to go to a chemist. If possible, sit in a warm bath until the symptoms have eased. Passing urine in the bath relieves a lot of the pain and is quite harmless, even if unorthodox! If taking a bath is not practicable, put your feet up or lie down and get some rest. See your doctor if:

● The attack lasts for more than 48 hours

● Attacks are frequent

● There is blood in your urine

● You are pregnant (the risk of kidney infection is serious)

To help prevent repeat attacks try to remove the cause. If you think there is infection, pay scrupulous attention to genital hygiene and get your partner to do the same. Wipe your bottom from front to back. If you think the cause is over-vigorous intercourse, find gentler ways of making love for a while and use a lubricant like KY jelly. If attacks seem to follow periods of stress and over-tiredness, the answer might be a holiday or at least a few days' rest.

Cancers_____

Like many forms of cancer, those affecting the reproductive organs can be prevented if they're caught in time. Regular checking for breast cancer and cancer of the testes, and screening for cancer of the cervix, is essential.

BREAST CANCER

Breasts have two reasons for existing: they have erotic appeal, and they feed offspring. They undergo enormous changes throughout life. All breasts are uneven in texture; you may mistake this unevenness for danger signs, but becoming familiar with your breasts will help you spot changes. Feeling your breasts regularly for any unusual swellings or lumps is easy to do with practice.

The best time is in the week after a period, because before and during a period the breasts are often lumpier than usual. The first thing to do is to stand in front of a mirror with your arms by your sides and look at the form and outline of your breasts.

● Are they the same size and shape?

● Is there any swelling, dimpling or puckering of the skin?

● Any rash or change of colour?

● Any discharge from the nipples? (A colourless fluid is quite normal.)

● Are nipples turning inwards having not been inverted previously?

Next, raise your arms above your head so that you can check underneath your breasts for the same signs.

The next step is to feel your breasts. This is best done on your back, either in the bath or lying flat on a bed with a towel or pillow under your shoulders.

1 Hunch your left shoulder and feel the left breast with the right hand. Flatten your fingers and press gently.

2 Working in a circular movement, start from the nipple and work outwards feeling for any thickening of the skin, swellings or lumps.

3 With your left arm above your head, elbow bent, circle again slowly, this time from outside to inside.

4 Finish by following the breastline up to the armpit to check the tail of the breast.

Repeat for the right breast.

If you find anything peculiar during the course of your investigations, report to your doctor as soon as you can. In the vast majority of cases of odd lumps found, the cause is traced to a cyst or non-cancerous growth which is easily cured.

CANCER OF THE CERVIX

Although this is still a rare condition, the number of women, particularly younger women, who are registered as having cancer of the cervix has been increasing recently. No one is sure why. It may be that the disease is being detected earlier and more often, so that fewer cases go undiscovered.

The herpes virus, earlier sex and more partners all appear to put women at greater risk of contracting cervical cancer, but there is now very strong evidence that the genital wart virus, which is proving more and more difficult to treat, may also be responsible. This would explain why women with several partners are more at risk than women with only one; the more partners the more likely it is that one of them will have warts on his penis. But it's important to remember that something like six out of ten women with cancer of the cervix have only ever had one partner. If the one person you have sex with has himself had several partners, he'll be that much more likely to have come into contact with the wart virus. If cancer of the cervix is traceable back to a virus carried by the penis, then barrier methods of contraception — the sheath or the cap — are extra-valuable.

Cervical cancer can take up to fifteen years to develop into full-blown cancer. In the early stages all that happens is that cells in the cervix begin to behave oddly; if a small smear sample of cervical tissue is examined under a microscope the changes can easily be detected.

A cervical smear or Pap test can be carried out in family planning clinics or by your family doctor. A tiny sample of tissue is smeared gently from the cervix with a small spatula or swab of cotton wool. This is quite painless. It is sent off to a laboratory and, in the unlikely event that there is anything wrong, the cancerous cells can be removed. IF a test is 'positive', it does not necessarily mean that there is cancer present. Cervical cells can also look abnormal if there is infection present. Further tests will sort this out.

Women should have one smear test carried out as soon as they start to have sex, and repeat tests at three year intervals. If you began to have intercourse at an early age, or have many partners, then ideally you should be tested once a year.

CANCER OF THE PENIS OR TESTICLES

These are fairly rare conditions, but like most cancers are best treated if detected early. Any inflammation, difficulty in passing urine, discharge, swelling, lump or pain in the penis or testicles should be reported to the doctor as soon as you notice it.

Useful Addresses

1. General information, advice and help

ADAM AND EVE COUNSELLING CENTRE
4 Merchant Quay
DUBLIN 8
Tel 0001 711910
Full counselling service

BRITISH ASSOCIATION FOR COUNSELLING
37a Sheep Street
RUGBY CV21 3BX
Tel (0788) 78328
Information about counselling services in Britain, mainly related to personal relationships and psycho-sexual problems. They also refer people who write or phone in

CITIZENS ADVICE BUREAU
Myddleton House
115-123 Pentonville road
LONDON N1 9LZ
Tel 01 833 2181
Free and confidential advice on a wide range of subjects. Contact this central address for your local branch

NATIONAL ASSOCIATION FOR YOUNG PERSONS' COUNSELLING AND ADVISORY SERVICES (NAYPCAS)
17-23 Albion Street
LEICESTER LE1 66D
Tel (0533) 554775
National information centre providing counselling, advice and information for young people

NATIONAL COUNCIL FOR CIVIL LIBERTIES
21 Tabard Street
LONDON SE1
Tel 01 403 3888
Free and confidential information on a wide range of subjects

NATIONAL MARRIAGE GUIDANCE COUNCIL
Herbert Gray College
Little Church Street
RUGBY
Warwickshire CV21 3AP
Appointments and counselling for married and single people in need of counselling

NEW GRAPEVINE
416 St John Street
LONDON EC1V 4NJ
Tel 01 278 9147
Advice and counselling for under 25s

STUDENTS NIGHTLINE
BANGOR Wales
Tel (0248) 2121
24-hour counselling service

STUDENTS NIGHTLINE
ABERDEEN Scotland
Tel (0224) 20909
Counselling, advice and activities for young people

WOMEN'S THERAPY CENTRE
6 Manor Gardens
LONDON N7
Tel 01 263 6200
Offers individual and group therapy and workshops

2. Emotional and sexual problems

THE ALBANY TRUST
24 Chester Square
LONDON SW1
Tel 01 730 5871
Free counselling for sexual and relationship problems

CAMPAIGN FOR HOMOSEXUAL EQUALITY
274 Upper Street
Islington LONDON N1
Tel 01 359 3973
A campaign organisation concerned with lobbying for homosexual rights. They publish books and free advice leaflets, but enclose an SAE when writing

FAMILY PLANNING INFORMATION SERVICE
27-35 Mortimer Street
LONDON W1
Tel 01 636 7866
Advice by phone or letter on psycho-sexual problems, referral to specialist organisations

GAY SWITCHBOARD
BM Switchboard
LONDON WC1N 3XX

Tel 01 837 7324

*24-hour confidential telephone
service for both men and women*

INCEST CRISIS LINE
66 Marriott Close
BEDFONT
Middlesex TW14 9PZ

Tel 01 890 4732

*Emergency helpline for incest victims.
Male and female telephone
counselling. Nationwide service
includes referral to specialist help
agencies. Phone or write for local
number*

**LONDON CENTRE FOR
PSYCHOTHERAPY**
19 Fitzjohns Avenue
LONDON NW3 5JY

Tel 01 435 0873

*Registered charity providing
counselling and individual or group
psychotherapy at moderate fees*

LONDON FRIEND
274 Upper Street
Islington LONDON N1

Tel 01 359 7371

*National network offering support,
advice and counselling to gay people
or to people who think they might be
gay*

RAPE CRISIS CENTRE
PO Box 69
LONDON WC1X 9NJ

Tel 01 278 3956 (office)
01 837 1600 (24 hour emergency)

*Free confidential service offering
counselling, medical and legal help
about rape and sexual assault
24 hours a day. Information about
sexually transmitted diseases, legal
and medical procedures, etc*

SAMARITANS
17 Uxbridge Road
SLOUGH Buckinghamshire

Tel 0753 32713

*Confidential 24-hour telephone
service for those in despair. Local
telephone numbers in telephone
directory*

SAPPHO
20 Dorset Square
LONDON NW1 6QB

Tel 01 724 3636

Support for gay women

**SEXUAL AND PERSONAL
RELATIONSHIPS OF THE
DISABLED (SPOD)**
286 Camden Road
LONDON N7 0BJ

Tel 01 607 8851

*Provides information, advice,
training, etc, about personal and
sexual rights of people with physical
or mental handicaps*

3. Birth control, pregnancy and abortion

**BRITISH PREGNANCY
ADVISORY SERVICE**
Austy Manor Wootten Wawen
SOLIHULL West Midlands

Tel 056 42 3225

*Non-profit-making charity offering
pregnancy tests, counselling, birth
control, pregnancy and abortion
advice. Local branches*

BROOK ADVISORY CENTRES
(Head Office)
153a East Street
LONDON SE17 2SD

Tel 01 708 1234

*National network of young people's
advisory centres. Completely
confidential pregnancy testing, birth
control advice and treatment, and
abortion counselling*

**FAMILY PLANNING
ASSOCIATION**
27-35 Mortimer Street
LONDON W1N 7RJ

Tel 01 636 7866

*Free enquiry service on all aspects of
sexuality and birth control. Wide
range of leaflets*

GINGERBREAD
35 Wellington Street
LONDON WC2

Tel 01 240 0953

*Help for one-parent families. Local
groups, activities, etc*

Useful Addresses

LIFE
7 The Parade
LEAMINGTON SPA
Warwickshire

Tel 0926 311677

Offers a pregnancy testing service, practical help and advice to pregnant women who opt not to have an abortion. Accommodation available for single women

NATIONAL COUNCIL FOR ONE PARENT FAMILIES
255 Kentish Town Road
LONDON NW5

Tel 01 267 1361

National campaigning body for one-parent families. Offers confidential advice and counselling to single pregnant women and single parents. Advice on legal and social problems

PREGNANCY ADVISORY SERVICES
11 Charlotte Street
LONDON W1P 1HD

Tel 01 637 8962

London-based centre of British Pregnancy Advisory Service

SCOTTISH COUNCIL FOR SINGLE PARENTS
13 Gayfield Square
EDINBURGH EH1 3NX

Tel 031 556 3899

Offers counselling for one-parent families

4. Health

HEALTH EDUCATION COUNCIL
78 New Oxford Street
LONDON WC1A 1AH

Tel 01 631 0930

Information on all aspects of health promotion. Free leaflets on sexually transmitted diseases, hygiene, personal relationships, etc

HERPES SELF HELP GROUP
41 North Road
LONDON N7

Tel 01 609 9061

Help for herpes sufferers and those who think they might be infected

Sexually Transmitted Disease Special Clinics

The address and nearest telephone number of your clinic can be found by ringing your local hospital or GP

TERRENCE HIGGINS TRUST
Helpline 01 278 8445

Advice and information on all aspects of AIDS

WOMEN'S HEALTH INFORMATION CENTRE
Ufton Centre
12 Ufton Road LONDON N1

Tel 01 251 6580

Reference library of articles on a variety of women's health topics

Index

Acknowledgements

Thanks to all FPA staff who helped with the book, including Zandria Pauncefort, Alastair Service, Helen Martins, Sue Ullrich, Ann Hodgson, Sharon Daniel, Charlotte Owen, Romie Goodchild and Ellen Bingham but especial thanks to Toni Belfield who not only did most of my work when I was writing the book, but also checked through the whole script with considerably more grace than her eleventh-hour deadline warranted.

Grateful thanks to Jane Harris for typing the manuscript and offering constructive comments. And thanks to all those people, young and not so young, who lent their opinions, comments and quotes — and sometimes even their faces.

PICTURE CREDITS

Family Planning Information Service 83, Tom Butler 77, 113, Posy Simmonds 61, 71 **The Image Bank** D Acomo 15 left, Jacques Alexandre 60 bottom, F Dardelet 145 top, R Farber 99, Zao-Grimberg 104, D Hamilton 94, 101, 121 bottom, E Herwig 159, Marcia Keegan 156, John Kelly 144-145, Ted Russell 38-39 **Multimedia Publications UK Limited** 11, 13, 14 right, 15 right, 16, 17 bottom, 18 middle, 22, 23, 35, 36, 37, 40 top right, 46 left, 47 bottom, 54 left, 55-57, 66 bottom, 69 inset, 70 middle, 81 bottom, 105, 106, 108, 110, 111 bottom, 117, 131, 133, 139, 141, 145 bottom, 146-147, 148, 149 bottom, 153, 154, 164-165, 168, 175, 179 **Multimedia/Chris Sowe** 7, 14 left, 18 top, 18 bottom, 21, 24-33, 45, 46 right, 49, 50-51, 82, 149 top, 152 top, 160, 161, 164 middle, 171, 173, 178 **Shari Peacock** contents, 6, 10, 20, 34, 52, 64, 66 top, 84, 96, 102-103, 116, 124-125, 130, 138, 143, 152, 166, 170, 174 **The Photo Source** 12, 17 top, 22-23, 36-37, 38 inset, 39, 47 top, 54 right, 67, 98, 154-155, 157, 158 **PictureBank** 61, 68, 114-115 **Professor Philip Rawson Collection** 134-135 **Relay Photos** 128 **Tony Stone Associates** 9, 19, 40 top left, 42, 43 top, 53, 118, 120, 121 top, 126-127, 177 **Errol Watson** 69, 78, 86-93, 109, 111 top, 112, 122, 123 **Zefa Picture Library** title, 8, 41 bottom, 43 bottom, 58, 60 top, 81 top, 85, 107, 119, 155, 162-163, 169

Front Cover: **Shari Peacock**
Back Cover: **Multimedia/Chris Sowe**

Multimedia Publications (UK) Limited have endeavoured to observe the legal requirements with regard to the suppliers of photographic material.